Sustainable Development Goals Series

The **Sustainable Development Goals Series** is Springer Nature's inaugural cross-imprint book series that addresses and supports the United Nations' seventeen Sustainable Development Goals. The series fosters comprehensive research focused on these global targets and endeavours to address some of society's greatest grand challenges. The SDGs are inherently multidisciplinary, and they bring people working across different fields together and working towards a common goal. In this spirit, the Sustainable Development Goals series is the first at Springer Nature to publish books under both the Springer and Palgrave Macmillan imprints, bringing the strengths of our imprints together.

The Sustainable Development Goals Series is organized into eighteen subseries: one subseries based around each of the seventeen respective Sustainable Development Goals, and an eighteenth subseries, "Connecting the Goals," which serves as a home for volumes addressing multiple goals or studying the SDGs as a whole. Each subseries is guided by an expert Subseries Advisor with years or decades of experience studying and addressing core components of their respective Goal.

The SDG Series has a remit as broad as the SDGs themselves, and contributions are welcome from scientists, academics, policymakers, and researchers working in fields related to any of the seventeen goals. If you are interested in contributing a monograph or curated volume to the series, please contact the Publishers: Zachary Romano [Springer; zachary.romano@springer.com] and Rachael Ballard [Palgrave Macmillan; rachael.ballard@palgrave.com].

Jodi Cressman • Lisa DeTora
Jeannie Ludlow • Nora Martin Peterson
Editors

Envisioning Embodiment in the Health Humanities

Interdisciplinary Approaches to Literature, Culture, and Media

palgrave
macmillan

Editors
Jodi Cressman
Dominican University
River Forest, IL, USA

Lisa DeTora
Hofstra University
South Hempstead, NY, USA

Jeannie Ludlow
Eastern Illinois University
Charleston, IL, USA

Nora Martin Peterson
University of Nebraska–Lincoln
Lincoln, NE, USA

ISSN 2523-3084 ISSN 2523-3092 (electronic)
Sustainable Development Goals Series
ISBN 978-3-031-49806-0 ISBN 978-3-031-49807-7 (eBook)
https://doi.org/10.1007/978-3-031-49807-7

This Palgrave Macmillan imprint is published by the registered company Springer Nature Switzerland AG.

The registered company address is: Gewerbestrasse 11, 6330 Cham, Switzerland

Paper in this product is recyclable.

Foreword

My interest in bodies began with the French Revolution. As I was researching a book on literary representations of the fall of the *ancien régime*, I grappled with two types of bodies. There were, on the one hand, allegorical personifications of political ideals such as liberty, tolerance, and republicanism and, on the other, individual physical bodies affected by the Revolution's social and political upheaval. Pouring over the wealth of primary and secondary sources, I soon realized that I was much less interested in the iconographic representation of Liberty as a female figure in a fluttering dress—a privileged topic in scholarship on the period—than in the depiction of the bodies of fictional characters and fictionalized historical figures. Late eighteenth and early nineteenth century authors staged the momentous change in the body politic as the story of an individual character's body. The bodies of their predominantly female protagonists all diverged, in one way or another, from the gender norms of their time. This is nowhere more visible than in those novels that portray the adventures of cross-dressed female soldiers on the battlefields of the French Revolutionary and Napoleonic wars.

After Judith Butler presented her theory of gender performativity in *Gender Trouble* (1990), she was asked the following question, which she quotes in her book *Bodies That Matter* (1993): "What about the materiality of the body, *Judy*?" (ix). Yes, indeed, what about the materiality of the body? I wondered, thinking about the bruised and battered bodies of cross-dressed soldiers, who dreaded the inquisitive eye of the battlefield surgeon more than the weapon of their opponent. There is no denying that we all inhabit a physical body that manifests itself through its materiality. And yet, the way we perceive this body is profoundly shaped by cultural constructions and performances. As Butler argues in response to her critics, the body is more than pre-cultural and pre-linguistic matter; it therefore matters to us, also beyond its materiality.

As I progressed in my work on the trials and tribulations of individual bodies during and after the French Revolution, I encountered medical textbooks that highlighted the body's constructed nature in an almost comically absurd way. In his *Anatomy of the Bones of the Human Body*, the early nineteenth-century scientist John Barclay included drawings that exaggerated those body parts that had emerged as the site for the political debate concerning gender roles: the skull and the pelvis. Barclay argued that sexual difference was found not only in the genitals but also in the entire human body. The female skeleton was depicted with an extremely narrow ribcage, a disproportionately small skull, and extraordinarily wide hips. In case his readers did not follow his argument, Barclay accompanied his illustration of the female skeleton with the picture of an ostrich and that of the male skeleton with the drawing of a horse. The illustration of the female skeleton begs the question about the real-life body serving as the model. It might have been a woman with unusually large hip bones and a small skull who was selected to highlight women's domestic destiny. Or it could have been, as cultural critic Londa Schiebinger ventures, the skeleton of a woman whose bones were deformed by decades of wearing a corset, which had squeezed her literally into her time's gender roles. Or, like the Greek painter Xeuxis (fifth century BC), the anatomist could have assembled the skeleton from several different women, each representing a specific body part in its supposed perfection. Bodies are not pre-cultural and pre-linguistic; they are constructed, shaped, and deformed by regulatory cultural ideals as well as individual desires.

The early nineteenth-century exaggeration of the differences between male and female bodies affirmed the very fact that anatomists strove to deny, namely that these bodies' commonalities by far exceeded their differences. The biological basis for the gender binary was questioned further by bodies hovering on the dividing line between male and female. As I was approaching the end of my project on French Revolutionary bodies, my question regarding gender and sexuality shifted from "What about the body?" to "What about the liminal body?" Ancient Greek mythology answered this question with the myth of Hermaphroditus. The son of Hermes and Aphrodite charms the nymph Salmacis to such a degree that she fuses her body with his, thereby creating neither the perfect male nor the perfect female but the perfect human form. Over the course of the past two millennia, the representation of this nonbinary body gradually changed from an image of perfect grace to that of a grotesque monster, and then, beginning in the early eighteenth century, to a mistake of nature in need of medical intervention. The eighteenth-century entry on the "hermaphrodite" in the *Encyclopédie,* the Enlightenment reference work par excellence, posited that the anatomist could classify this liminal body as either male or female. This normalizing tendency continued in subsequent centuries, only with different tools. The pen of the eighteenth-century *encyclopédiste* was replaced first with the microscope of the nineteenth-century scientist and then the scalpel of the twentieth-century surgeon. Only in the late twentieth and early twenty-first centuries did those whose bodies were normalized by the medical establishment speak out about their embodied experience and create activist organizations. The classification, scrutiny, and normalization of the nonbinary body highlights, in particularly powerful ways, the fact that bodies are contested realities embedded in their time's body politic.

My research on eighteenth-century hermaphrodites highlighted the fact that all embodied experience is liminal and changing.[1] The chapters in this volume propose to express some of these experiences, aware that accessing the embodied experience of others necessarily remains fragmentary and incomplete. Bodies matter and they do so in ways that defy disciplinary boundaries. The scholars in the present volume explore cultural sites ranging from seventeenth-century courtly handbooks to present-day Instagram posts where the experience of the self and others may be envisioned from a variety of perspectives. By mobilizing and putting into dialogue interpretive frameworks such as disability studies, comics studies, gender studies, health humanities, posthuman studies, rhetoric, and cultural studies, the authors in this volume demonstrate that bodies matter. Envisioning embodiment is an interdisciplinary practice that mobilizes intersectional identities of race, class, and gender and does so by giving

[1] See, for example, "Orientation and Supplementation: Locating the 'Hermaphrodite' in the *Encyclopédie.*" *Goethe Yearbook* 22 (July 2015): 169–187; "Enlightenment Angst: James Parsons' A Mechanical and Critical Enquiry into the Nature of Hermaphrodites (1741)." *Taking Stock: Twenty-Five Years of Comparative Literary Research.* Ed. Norbert Bachleitner, Achim Hölter, and John McCarthy (Leiden and Boston: Brill, 2020) 247–269; and "Epistemological Anxiety: The Case of Michel-Anne Drouart." *Intelligible States: Bodies and/as Transitions in the Health Humanities.* Co-edited with Lisa DeTora (London and New York: Routledge, 2019).

voice to the multiple ways in which embodied knowledge expresses itself. Bodies matter and theories of embodiment allow us to perceive the ways in which they do.

University of Illinois at Urbana-Champaign Stephanie M. Hilger

Bibliography

Butler, Judith. *Bodies That Matter: On the Discursive Limits of Sex*. Taylor and Francis, 1993.

———. *Gender Trouble: Feminism and the Subversion of Identity*. Routledge, 1990.

Barclay, John. *The Anatomy of the Bones of the Human Body: Represented in a Series of Engravings, Copied from the Elegant Tables of Sue & Albinus*. Engraver Edward Mitchell. Edinburgh: Maclachlan & Stewart, 1829.

"Hermaphrodite, sub. & adj. (Anat.)." In *Encyclopédie, ou dictionnaire raisonné des sciences, des arts et des métiers, etc.* University of Chicago: ARTFL Encyclopédie Project (Spring 2013 Edition). Ed. Robert Morrissey. http://encyclopedie.uchicago.edu/. Vol. 6. 165–167.

Hilger, Stephanie. "Orientation and Supplementation: Locating the 'Hermaphrodite' in the *Encyclopédie*." *Goethe Yearbook* 22 (July 2015): 169–187.

———. "Enlightenment Angst: James Parsons' *A Mechanical and Critical Enquiry into the Nature of Hermaphrodites* (1741)." *Taking Stock: Twenty-Five Years of Comparative Literary Research*. Ed. Norbert Bachleitner, Achim Hölter, and John McCarthy. Leiden and Boston: Brill, 2020. 247–269.

———. "Epistemological Anxiety: The Case of Michel-Anne Drouart." *Intelligible States: Bodies and/as Transitions in the Health Humanities*. Co-edited with Lisa DeTora. London and New York: Routledge, 2019. 22–34.

Schiebinger, Londa. *The Mind Has No Sex?: Women in the Origins of Modern Science*. Boston: Harvard University Press, 1991.

Contents

Notes on Contributors

Shalini Abayasekara is a graduate student at the Ohio State University. Shalini is in the Department of English's *Writing, Rhetoric, and Literacy* program and is just wrapping up her MA. Her main areas of interest are the rhetoric of health and medicine and disability studies. Within these fields, she is especially keen to consider the rhetorical nature of classification regarding health conditions, and how an individual diagnosed with an illness or disability views their own health-related experience. Before joining Ohio State's MA/PhD program, Shalini taught for 5.5 years at the University of Colombo, Sri Lanka.

Jodi Cressman is Professor of English at Dominican University, in River Forest, Illinois, where she teaches courses in contemporary literature, graphic narrative, creative writing, and the health humanities. Together with Lisa DeTora, she co-edited *Graphic Embodiments: Perspectives on Health and Embodiment in Graphic Narratives.* She has published essays on witnessing as an embodied act as well as on company and counterbalance in Ellen Forney's *Marbles.* She is working on a book-length creative project that explores the history of disasters in American towns named Centralia.

Lisa DeTora is Associate Professor and the Director of STEM Writing at Hofstra University, where she teaches courses in health communication, scientific writing, literary studies, rhetoric, and chemistry. Lisa's publishing includes co-edited volumes on embodiment with Jodi Cressman and Stephanie Hilger as well as work in comics studies, biomedical publication ethics, rhetoric of health and medicine, health communication and technical communication.

Derek Ettensohn is Associate Professor of English and the Humanities at Sewanee: The University of the South. He works in the fields of global Anglophone literature and the health humanities and is interested in the representation of illness and the ethics of care in film and the contemporary Anglophone novel. His work has appeared in journals such as *College Literature*, *Critique: Studies in Contemporary Fiction*, and *Modern Fiction Studies*.

Serena Fusco is Assistant Professor of Comparative Literature at the University of Naples "L'Orientale". Among her publications: the monographs *Incorporations of Chineseness: Hybridity, Bodies, and Chinese American Literature* (Cambridge Scholars Publishing, 2016) and *Confini porosi. Pelle e rappresentazione in quattro narrazioni della modernità* [Porous Borders: Skin and Representation in Four Narratives of Modernity] (Scripta, 2018). Her research is multilingual and transcultural in scope and includes Chineseness in the transnational space; East/West comparative literature and world literature; Asian American literature; intermediality, photography, and dialogues between literature and photography; and the internationalization of education.

Amanda K. Greene is a research specialist at the Center for Bioethics and Social Sciences in Medicine (CBSSM) at the University of Michigan Medical School. Her scholarship is invested in understanding social media as a social determinant of health, specifically investigating the roles it plays in both sustaining and dismantling health inequities. At CBSSM she focuses on research projects exploring women's representation in science and academic medicine, patient decision-making and experiences with chronic illness, as well as the ethical, legal, and social implications of health data sharing.

Barbara Grüning is Associate Professor of Sociology of Culture at the University of Milan-Bicocca. She is a member of the Research Committee on Comics and Graphic Narrative of the International Comparative Literature Association (ICLA) since its foundation in 2015. Her research areas concern the sociology of space, the sociology of body, the fields of cultural production, mental illness, the representation and spatialization of social phenomena in comics and other media and the relationship among comics, social theory and social research.

Stephanie M. Hilger is a scholar of eighteenth-century literature and culture, with a focus on gender studies and health humanities. She is Professor of German and Comparative Literature. In addition, she holds appointments in the European Union Center, French, and Gender and Women's Studies. Since 2021, she has also been affiliated with the Department of Biomedical and Translational Sciences at the Carle Illinois College of Medicine. In addition to her monographs (*Liminal Bodies*, 2024; *Gender and Genre*, 2014; and *Women Write Back*, 2009), she has (co-)edited four volumes in the health humanities: *The Bloomsbury Handbook to the Health Humanities in German Studies* (2024); *Bodies and Transitions in the Health Humanities: Intelligible States of Corporeality* (with Lisa DeTora, 2019); *New Directions in Literature and Medicine Studies* (2017); and *The Early History of Embodied Cognition from 1740 to 1920* (with John McCarthy, Nicholas Saul, and Heather Sullivan, 2015).

Elizabeth Lanphier is an assistant professor in the Ethic Center at Cincinnati Children's Hospital Medical Center and the Department of Pediatrics in the University of Cincinnati College of Medicine. She is also affiliated faculty in the University of Cincinnati Departments of Philosophy; Women, Gender, and Sexuality Studies; and the Center for Public Engagement with Science; and is a non-resident research fellow with the Institute for Philosophy and Public Policy. Elizabeth holds a master's degree in Narrative Medicine from Columbia University and a PhD in Philosophy from Vanderbilt University, where she also completed a post-doctoral fellowship in Clinical Ethics.

Jeannie Ludlow is Professor of English and Director of Women's, Gender, and Sexuality Studies at Eastern Illinois University. She has worked as an abortion patient advocate and an anti-racist advocate and trainer. Her research interests include representations of abortion and reproduction in contemporary literature and writing, abortion discourse, and activist pedagogy. Recent publications include "Full Bleed: The Graphic Period at the End of the Menstrual Narrative," in *Graphic Perspectives on Health and Embodiment*, edited by Cressman and DeTora (Leuven University Press, 2021); and "It's A ~~Boy!~~borted: Visualizing the Fetus in Abortion Narratives," in *Representing Abortion*, edited by Rachel Hurst (Routledge, 2021).

Nora Martin Peterson is Associate Professor of French Cultural Studies at the University of Nebraska-Lincoln. She is the author of *Involuntary Confessions of the Flesh in Early Modern France* (Delaware, 2016), and editor of *Miracles of Love: French Fairy Tales by Women* (MLA, 2021). She has published articles on Michel de Montaigne, Marguerite de Valois, Marguerite de Navarre, and the *Princesse de Clèves*. Her research, broadly defined, focuses on early modern literature and culture, with particular interests in women's writing; the body; health humanities, and intersections between literature and religion, legal history and courtly handbooks.

Kaitlyn Waller is an independent scholar. She received her MA in Modern Languages & Literatures from the University of Nebraska-Lincoln in 2022. Her research explores the intersections of migration narratives and young adult literature, with a particular focus on francophone authors. She has worked in international education for over a decade, holding positions in the United States, France, China, and (most recently) South Korea. Kaitlyn has a Masters of French Studies from the University of Wisconsin- Madison (2016) and a Bachelor's degree in French from Grinnell College (2013).

Sophie Witt is Professor of Literary Studies, Knowledge Cultures, and Interdisciplinarity at the University of Hamburg; she was Assistant Professor in Literary and Theatre Studies at the German Department of the University of Zurich, and an associate member of the Zurich-based Center of the History of Knowledge and part of its Medical Humanities Working Group. She wrote her second book on the relation of theatricality and psychosomatics with a five-year PRIMA grant from the Swiss National Science Foundation.

List of Figures

PART I

Envisioning the Self

Introduction: Envisioning Embodiment

Jodi Cressman, Lisa DeTora, Jeannie Ludlow, and Nora Martin Peterson

Introduction

Our work originates in the idea of humility, a concept with a strong linkage to health humanities through Sayantani Das Gupta's conception of narrative humility (2008). Das Gupta traces this concept from origins in two different intellectual threads. The first, cultural humility, derives from

J. Cressman (✉)
Dominican University, River Forest, IL, USA
e-mail: jcressman@dom.edu

L. DeTora
Hofstra University, South Hempstead, NY, USA
e-mail: Lisa.M.DeTora@hofstra.edu

J. Ludlow
Eastern Illinois University, Charleston, IL, USA
e-mail: jludlow@eiu.edu

N. Martin Peterson
University of Nebraska–Lincoln, Lincoln, NE, USA
e-mail: npeterson10@unl.edu

J. Cressman et al. (eds.), *Envisioning Embodiment in the Health Humanities*, Sustainable Development Goals Series,
https://doi.org/10.1007/978-3-031-49807-7_1

anthropological studies and relies on accepting the impossibility of cultural competence, which assumed an ability to master outside cultures. The second, narrative medicine, draws its power from actively seeking out, listening to, and valuing, stories of illness. Each of these threads can be understood as multifaceted, multidisciplinary attempts to understand something outside the self. Narrative humility depends on a recognition of the impossibility of ever fully understanding the experience of another, yet remaining engaged in the endeavor, nevertheless. This type of humility informs the chapters that comprise the current volume. We seek to understand various aspects of embodiment as it intersects with an interplay of language and image or envisioning that is often necessary to imagine the experiences of others. We acknowledge that full understanding may be impossible, but like Das Gupta, we believe the attempt remains valuable and necessary.

Our chapters operate within a broader discourse of embodiment that can be linked back to the emergence of posthumanity, which recognizes inherent problems in conceptualizing embodied experience. Donna Haraway (1991) troubled the differences among human, animal, and machine, highlighting the imprecise and blurred boundaries between these categories, hence any category that can be used to define embodied experience. Judith Butler (1990, 1993, 2004, 2008), drawing on Michel Foucault, also noted that embodied experiences must enter a symbolic realm, like language, to exist as knowledge. But language has only a limited ability to capture embodied experiences, particularly those that separate individuals and groups. Something will always be lost in this translation, no matter how many people believe they share certain experiences. Elaine Scarry (1985), for instance, notes that the near-universal phenomenon of pain is never fully sharable. The pain of others is always imagined in connection to our own personal histories.

The chapters collected here use various theoretical models to forward conversations about embodiment and to make embodied experiences legible and meaningful to outsiders. Of note, narrative humility is currently a commonplace of health humanities, an indispensable conceptual framework. Yet, as Emily Heavey (2015) notes, narrative constrains an understanding of embodied experience in all disciplines. We, like Heavey, consider that envisioning embodiment can begin to address the incompleteness of most accounts of embodied experience.

Envisioning Embodiment

The idea that envisioning can be used to fill in gaps between knowledge and embodied experiences draws on Carlyle's notion that visualizing creates mental and abstract images of ideas (cf. Kleege 2015). When faced with partial or incomplete ideas, a reader often fills in the gaps, imagining the remainder. Discourse has its own material properties, through which we make sense of lived experiences, which suggests that embodied experience is never fully separate or primary. The tendency to allow discourses, or knowledge, to overtake embodied experience requires resistance and attention to various types of study. For instance, the work of scholars like Butler, Anne Fausto-Sterling (2012) and Suzanne Kessler (1998) attempted to decouple biology from cultural ideas about sex, reinforcing the fact that embodied characteristics like race and gender are performed. Gender, however, is only one way of understanding embodied experience (cf. DeTora and Hilger, 2020).

Disability studies troubles the fiction of a Platonically whole, integrated body (see Adams et al. 2015) as well as the means of filling in the gaps between knowledge and experience. What Georgina Kleege (2015) calls "visuality" (176), or how society uses visual culture to reinforce unhelpful visions of disabled persons, indicates the dangers of unbridled thought. As Abby Wilkerson (2015) notes, disability studies tends to reject the linkage of "embodiment" (71) with "corporeality" (71), instead emphasizing personal subjectivity. Such an accounting must be envisioned to be understood, even as narrative humility will emphasize that an ongoing move toward better understanding will never be complete. The related field of trauma studies, with its focus on specific incidents and transformational moments, can open or forestall an understanding of certain types of embodied experience (see Balaev 2012). Here again, understanding might, or must, remain partial and incomplete because of the need to unpack, analyze and examine a moment of trauma that resists an entry into the realm of knowledge. Returning to Butler (1993), one might see the operation of abjection or unlivable elements of embodied experience.

One potentially helpful construct for bridging embodied, yet unspoken experiences with knowledge comes from comics studies. Thierry Groensteen (1999/2011) presented a system that accounted for the synergies between text, images, and gaps on and across pages. Comics may draw attention to the ways readers participate in creating a whole out of segments. This interplay of visual and textual culture has been offered as a site where the unspeakable may inform intellectual discourses by scholars like Hilary Chute (2016, 2017), Hannah Miodrag (2015), and Elizabeth El Refaie (2019). Graphic Medicine (c.f., Czerwiec et al. 2015), a field with strong ties to the health humanities, has embraced the potential for comic books and graphic narratives to render experiences more legible even if they cannot be spoken.

No one solution exists to the problem of bridging embodied experience and the exchange of knowledge, particularly when thinking through the connection between narrative forms and lived experience. Various theories of hybridity, of prosthesis, of augmentation tell us that the very heart of embodied experience and personal identity are never fully knowable to another. Narrative humility helps us to understand that intersectional identities, which as Kimberlé Crenshaw (2005) has observed only compound the difficulties of communication and understanding, necessitate an enhanced attention to, and respect for, the thoughts and words of others. The work of feminist theorists, from Audre Lorde (1984) and the Combahee River Collective in the 1970s through the paradigm-shifting *This Bridge Called My Back* (1981/2015) to more recent work by Patricia Hill Collins (2006), M. Jacqui Alexander, (2006) Chela Sandoval (2008), and bell hooks (2013), has expanded critiques of embodiment. These thinkers have interrogated the ways racialization has been used to exclude Black people, indigenous people, and people of color from historically and culturally constructed categories of human embodiment. However, as Crenshaw reminds us, the nuances of personal identity become more complicated when layered.

Envisioning Embodiment in the Health Humanities

The visual dimensions of technological and scientific challenges presented by contemporary and historical practices remains an underexamined discourse within the broader vantage point of the health humanities. Similar limitations may be observed in rhetorical studies of embodiment or graphic medicine, suggesting that further work is needed to address how visual culture impacts our understanding of embodied experiences. In recognition of the fact that embodied materiality shifts through both interactions and time, health humanities offers a responsive approach to arts, humanities, and interpretation. Health humanities is capacious, opening space for the perspectives of patients and their loved ones, caregivers, health care providers, and practitioners and teachers of wellness, as the diverse analyses and interpretations in this volume demonstrate.

These chapters are situated in relationship to the "burgeoning field" of health humanities (Purser, qtd. in Crawford et al. 2020, 1). Evolving from the field of medical humanities, health humanities is perhaps best understood as an epistemology aiming to "advanc[e] health care, health and well-being" (Crawford et al. 2020, 3) through practical consideration of the materiality of the body. A rich interdisciplinary field, health humanities arose from the desire to humanize medicine and "create knowledgeable and sensitive health care providers, patients, and family caregivers" (Klugman, qtd. in Klugman and Lamb 2019). While medical humanities sought to "instill humanistic values in the physician," health humanities' broader focus reflects awareness that "health is more than just medicine" and that "the field of health belongs to everyone" (Klugman and Lamb 2019). In the introduction to *The Routledge Companion to Health Humanities* (2020), Paul Crawford (2015) characterizes the newer field as inclusive, democratizing, and applied, combining methods and knowledges from medical humanities with arts and public arts to "advance creative public health." This characterization builds on Crawford's and colleagues' earlier description in *Health Humanities* (in Crawford 2015), which links healthcare and humanities through modes of meaning-making ascribed to both fields. Similar epistemological overlaps recur in allied fields like narrative medicine. In carving out these terrains, authors and practitioners discovered vast potential cross-fertilizations yet to be unearthed, even as their work gained traction across multiple disciplines. In their chapter on inter- and transdisciplinarity in health humanities, Christian Riegel and Katherine M. Robinson note that analyses and interpretations in health humanities, "even when … practised with a disciplinary focus," are situated along the "contours of interdisciplinarity and transdisciplinarity" (2023, 176). This situatedness, they suggest, provides a strong foundation for dismantling the "theory-application divide" (188).

While health humanities has a well-deserved reputation as a practical and practicable set of applications that expand our empathy for embodied experiences, these chapters in particular are interested in those spaces or moments when embodiment exceeds understanding—when it becomes difficult for you to comprehend my experience—and the attempts we make to bridge that empathic gap. We think of these gaps and our attempts to reach across them in terms of envisioning. "Envisioning" has two common meanings: narrowly defined, it denotes an ability to see; more broadly, it implies imagination. Envisioning embodiment, then, describes what we can try to do together when it becomes difficult for you to comprehend my experience. As I work to make my experience more apprehendable to you, you can work to see it more clearly or to imagine it. Together, we are engaged in a dynamic of representation and interpretation that typifies humanities scholarship, broadly conceived. In the process, we may also become more consciously aware of just how elusive is full comprehension of another's embodied experiences.

Responding to the gaps that shape and interrupt our comprehension of embodiment, the individual chapters collected here focus on diverse hybrid and prosthetic experiences. Considered in conversation with one another, they suggest that studying different kinds of incompleteness can underpin an ability to envision embodiment integratively. Building on "the magic of health humanities" (Crawford et al. 2020, 3) to welcome a diversity of perspectives, encourage collaboration between and among theories, methods, and expertises, and challenge hierarchies of knowledge (Crawford et al. 2020, 3–4), this volume eschews definitive conclusions. Rather, it proceeds from the belief that tensions inherent in reading multiple partial experiences can yield opportunities for hybrid knowledge-production. Thus, the chapters collected in this volume seek to interrogate the idea that the experiences of others are never knowable and to analyze cultural sites where the experiences of others may be envisioned by various means. We see the liminal and often incomplete places where these imaginings take shape as fruitful points of inquiry for representing seemingly unshareable sites of knowledge. The current volume examines the ways in which these imaginings inform our ideas (and ideals) of embodied knowledge, particularly as they intersect with current conversations and lived experience. Individual chapters explore embodied discourses as increasingly embedded in social and textual network across various media.

The stakes of these conversations extend beyond intellectual inquiry. Our volume and its individual contributions promote greater understanding that can support various of the United Nations' Sustainable Development Goals (SDGs) (17 Goals 2023). We also believe that goals such as quality education (SDG 4), gender equality (SDG 5), good health and well-being (SDG 3) have the potential to inform the questions our authors consider. Work that investigates the relationships between health, the humanities, and visual culture also has the potential to support peace, justice, and strong institutions (SDG 17), especially when one considers the pedagogical, performative, and activist turns of some of the contributions.

Our Volume

The foreword by Stephanie Hilger lays out a research trajectory that illustrates the historical importance of understanding persons with intersex bodies. In the eighteenth century, specific high-profile cases set the stage for determining the bounds of binary gender constructs For Hilger, this study "highlighted the fact that all embodied experience is liminal and changing," the location of this observation at the emergence of current understandings of gender provides a launching point for additional observations. We divided the main portion of this volume into two parts: "Envisioning the Self" and "Envisioning the Other."

Chapters in "Envisioning the Self," interrogate how visual technologies may enhance or participate in the epistemology of embodied experience. These authors take up a wide-ranging array of representations, analyzing texts and images produced across five centuries and several genres, from dramatic fiction to memoir and visual self-representation. These texts also analyze materials produced with both prescriptive and descriptive authorial intent. The chapters in "Envisioning the Self" illustrate how these varied and diverse texts each focus on how visual technologies enhance narratives of embodied experience by destabilizing notions of completeness and simultaneously providing information that helps complete obvious gaps. Chapters in the subsequent section, "Envisioning the Other," consider how othering can circumscribe engagement with technologies that construct visual representations of the self. These chapters consider work that illustrates how a desire for embodied coherence always exists in tension with an inability to fully imagine the embodied coherence of others. This tension provides an infrastructure within which we turn to technologies of envisioning.

Envisioning the Self

The two opening chapters in Part 1, Nora Martin Peterson's "Filling in the Gaps: Fragments, Scripts, and Gender in Early Modern France" and Sophie Witt's "Theatres of Psychosomatics," present early modern technologies of envisioning embodiment. Peterson's chapter reads prescriptive courtly handbooks alongside the memoirs of the Abbé de Choisy, considering how people shape and curate self-representations in the service of embodied coherence. Witt's focus on an eighteenth-century play provides insight into psychosomatics, which emerged as a way to understand embodied coherence within a specific context of illness. Serena Fusco's "Reappropriating Breastfeeding as Power and Time in Photography and Feminist Discourse" then presents a contemporary example of how technologies can be intentionally deployed to document and defend individual choices. As Fusco discusses, photoprojects about breastfeeding strategically mobilize partial or veiled images to challenge the notion that breastfeeding is always a private choice about a private act.

The following chapters consider largely invisible and psychological phenomena. Amanda Greene in "Enactment, Entanglement, #Endometriosis: Feminist Technoscience and the Instagrammatic Illness Narrative," reads Instagram posts about endometriosis as examples of what narrative medicine and health humanities experts would call wounded storytelling. In their Instagram posts, users employ visual technology to represent their illness experience as a critical component of selfhood. In this context, endometriosis, which is often questioned as a legitimate or authentic medical experience, can be rendered visible to others. Greene takes up an explicitly health humanistic perspective to interpret work that is often also considered from positions of visual rhetoric or technical communication. Similarly, in "Narrating Anorexia in Graphic Novels: A Body-Space Analysis" Barbara Grüning focuses on visual representations of invisible illnesses commonly understood to disrupt embodied cohesion. Grüning examines how graphic narratives about eating disorders represent self-perception among people with anorexia and bulimia experience, integrating questions about health and illness within a frame of social science inquiry that provides a foil to Greene's intellectual and theoretical framing. Finally, Elizabeth Lanphier's "Rehearsing Grief: Turning to Look at Loss in *Eurydice*" considers Sara Ruhl's 2003 play, emphasizing the power of theatre in teaching audiences to reframe experiences of grief. Framing the analysis through Wittgenstein, Lanphier also offers a means of bridging the intellectual discourses within this volume with philosophical work.

Envisioning the Other

Derek Ettensohn in "'Why Should I Imagine Such a Thing?': Suffering in Michael Haneke's *Amour*," like Lanphier, challenges the reader to consider the limitations of empathy and an ability to envision ourselves and/in others. "The Myth of France: Identity Construction Through Migration in Young Adult Francophone Literature" by Kaitlyn Waller, maps out problems of identity formation in francophone narratives of migration. By analyzing texts from the twentieth and twenty-first centuries, Waller shows how personal identities and national identifications can be entwined and mutually influential. In "Making the Rounds: Information, Belief, and Breath in Alice Walker's 'Strong Horse Tea,'" Jodi Cressman turns to a1973 short story as a window for understanding the deadly consequences of racial disparities in health care. Cressman goes on to analyze institutional failures to envision the needs of marginalized populations, showing the deep relationship of othering and health disparities in literature and culture. Lisa DeTora's "The Mythology You Built: *After Forever's* Narrative of Visual Desire," examines another site of othering that can influence viewers' abilities to envision new ways of understanding. *After Forever*, DeTora posits, presents a novel version of queer melancholia that reintegrates closeted identities, the AIDS crisis and post-antiretroviral medical interventions in an age of legal gay marriage.

Two chapters take up questions of embodiment and representation during the recent pandemic. Shalini Abayasekara considers recent problems of embodied experience and grief during the COVID-19 pandemic in Sri Lanka. In "Dead Matter: COVID-19 and the Banning of Burials in Sri Lanka," Abayasekara maps out tensions that arise from othering specific ethnic and religious groups during times of crisis. The volume concludes with Jeannie Ludlow's chapter, "Vaccinated by the Blood: Antiabortion Mobilization of the COVID Body." Ludlow analyzes how antiabortion protesters embodied strategies of dominance and othering at a prochoice rally. By leveraging vaccination status and the dangers COVID infections, these antiabortion groups physically intimidated and dominated prochoice demonstrators by threatening their health. In the shift from perceiving others as threats to making physical threats, protesters embody a future in which technologies of envisioning and their significance to selves and others will continue to shape the personal and the political.

Overall, the volume's multiplicity seeks to replicate an essential and underlying truth of embodiment: if incompleteness can be an act of self-creation, then exploring many kinds of incompleteness side by side makes that act richer and more authentic to the acts of approximation involved in the human experience. Another feature that makes the volume unique is its approach of bringing together chapters that focus on connections between fiction and nonfiction. Both modes inform the field of health humanities in different ways; bringing them together here provides the opportunity for synergy and comparative readings. As such, the discourses approach embodiment from a variety of modes of inquiry and provide a variety of complementary frameworks. We sincerely hope that this collection enriches the intellectual domain of embodiment studies.

Bibliography

Adams, Rachel, et al., editors. *Keywords for Disability Studies.* NYU Press, 2015.

Alexander, M. Jacqui. *Pedagogies of Crossing: Meditations on Feminism, Sexual Politics, Memory, and the Sacred.* Duke University Press, Combined Academic, 2006.

Balaev, Michelle. *The Nature of Trauma in American Novels.* Northwestern UP, 2012.

Butler, Judith. *Bodies That Matter: On the Discursive Limits of Sex.* Taylor and Francis, 1993.

Butler, Judith. *Gender Trouble: Feminism and the Subversion of Identity.* Routledge, 1990.

Butler, Judith. *Giving an Account of Oneself.* Fordham UP, 2008.

Butler, Judith. *Undoing Gender.* Routledge, 2004.

Chute, Hilary. *Disaster Drawn: Visual Witness, Comics, and Documentary Form.* Harvard UP, 2017.

Chute, Hilary. *Why Comics? From Underground to Everywhere.* Harper Collins, 2016.

Collins, Patricia Hill. *Black Sexual Politics: African Americans, Gender, and the New Racism.* Routledge, 2006.

Combahee River Collective (2015). "A Black Feminist Statement." *This Bridge Called My Back*, 4th edition, SUNY Press, pp. 234–44.

Crawford, Paul, et al., editors. *Health Humanities*, Palgrave Macmillan, 2015.

Crawford, Paul, et al., editors. *The Routledge Companion to the Health Humanities*, Routledge, 2020.

Crenshaw, Kimberlé. (2005). "Mapping the Margins: Intersectionality, Identity Politics, and Violence against Women of Color (1994)." *Violence against women: Classic papers*, edited by R. K. Bergen, J. L. Edleson, and C. M. Renzetti, Pearson Education New Zealand, pp 282–313.

Czerwiec, MK, et al. *Graphic Medicine Manifesto.* Penn State University Press, 2015.

Das Gupta Sayatani. "Narrative humility." *Lancet.* 2008 Vol. 371 No. 9617; pp 980–1. https://doi.org/10.1016/s0140-6736(08)60440-7.

DeTora, Lisa, and Stephanie M. Hilger, editors. *Bodies in Transition in the Health Humanities: Representations of Corporeality.* Routledge, 2020.

El Refaie, Elisabeth. *Visual Metaphor and Embodiment in Graphic Illness Narratives.* Oxford UP, 2019.

Fausto-Sterling, Anne. *Sex/Gender: Biology in a Social World*. Routledge, 2012.
Groensteen, Thierry. *System of Comics*. Translated by Ann Miller. U of Mississippi P, 2011. Originally published as: *Systeme de la bande desinee* (1999).
Haraway, Donna J. *Simians, Cyborgs, and Women: The Reinvention of Nature*. Routledge, 1991.
Heavey, Emily. "Narrative Bodies, Embodied Narratives." *The Handbook of Narrative Analysis*, edited by Anna De Fina and Alexandra Georgakopoulou, Wiley Blackwell, 2015.
hooks, bell. *Writing beyond Race: Living Theory and Practice*. Routledge, 2013.
Kessler, Suzanne J. *Lessons from the Intersexed*. Rutgers, 1998.
Kleege, Georgina. "Visuality." *Keywords for Disability Studies*, edited by Rachel Adams, et al., NYU Press, 2015, pp. 176–177.
Klugman, Craig M., and Erin Gentry Lamb. "Introduction: Raising Health Humanities." *Research Methods in Health Humanities*, edited by alibris ebook, 2019.
Lorde, Audre. *Sister Outsider: Essays and Speeches*. Crossing Press, 1984.
Miodrag, Hannah. *Comics and Language: Reimagining Critical Discourse on the Form*. UP of Mississippi, 2015.
Moraga, Cherríe, and Gloria E. Anzaldúa. *This Bridge Called My Back: Writings by Radical Women of Color*, 4th edition. SUNY Press, 2015.
Riegel, Christian, and Katherine M. Robinson. "Interdisciplinarity, Transdisciplinarity, and Health Humanities: Eye Tracking, Ableism, Disability, and Art Creation." *Health Humanities in Application*, edited by Christian Reigel and Katherin M. Robinson. Palgrave Macmillan, 2023, pp. 175–93.
Sandoval, Chela. *Methodology of the Oppressed*. Foreword by Angela Y. Davis. Univ. of Minnesota Press, 2008.
Scarry, Elaine. *The Body in Pain: The Making and Unmaking of the World*. Oxford UP, 1985.
"The 17 Goals | Sustainable Development." *United Nations Department of Economic and Social Affairs* (2023), sdgs.un.org/goals. Accessed 31 May 2023.
Wilkerson, Abby. *Keywords for Disability Studies*, edited by Rachel Adams, et al., NYU Press, 2015.

Filling in the Gaps: Fragments, Scripts, and Gender in Early Modern France

Nora Martin Peterson

Introduction

When Baldassare Castiglione's *The Book of the Courtier* first appeared in 1528, it spread like wildfire to the courts and readers of Europe. Framed as a discussion about a hypothetical courtier by a group of noble interlocutors, it outlines the ideal traits, behaviors, and education of a courtier so that he might best serve his prince. Success in the world of the courtier depends largely on creating an embodied performance: "The Courtier must take great care to make a good impression at the start, and consider how damaging and fatal a thing it is to do otherwise" (Castiglione 2002, 2.36:97).[1] In early modern century Europe, prescriptive handbooks played a central role in the body politic, shaping behaviors,

[1] All citations from Castiglione's text will be noted in following order and format: book. chapter.page.

N. Martin Peterson (✉)
University of Nebraska–Lincoln, Lincoln, NE, USA
e-mail: npeterson10@unl.edu

J. Cressman et al. (eds.), *Envisioning Embodiment in the Health Humanities*, Sustainable Development Goals Series,
https://doi.org/10.1007/978-3-031-49807-7_2

conversations, and the way that people interacted with one another at court. Articulating everything from background and education to dress and conversation, these handbooks regulated many aspects of self-representation, and created what Harry Berger Jr. has called "a technology of behavioral performance" (Berger Jr. 2002, 295). In the early modern period, most courtly handbooks were written for men, prescribing and defining masculinity via a series of textual performances. However, the tight focus on how individuals inhabited their social roles applies to constructions of how people thought about gender and self-representation outside the context of courtly handbooks, as well. As Lewis Seifert writes (2009), "in the history of early modern science, … the sexed body was (re)conceptualized during this period" (3). Kathleen Long indicates (2006) that early modern medicine was aware of the "gap … between the surface presentations of gender, and … underlying structures; these two aspects of a person may even contradict each other" (80). Long continues that for seventeenth-century French surgeon Jacques Duval, "visual cues of gender are linked to performative presentations (dress, speech, gesture, comportment, etc.); touch is linked to the underlying body, which he considers more 'essential' or more 'real' than the surface presentations" (105). The (limited) freedom to invent and problematize the boundaries of gender is important to reconsidering early modern discussions of gender. Of particular interest is the extent to which early modern bodies can be grounded in a framework of embodiment that relies on fragmentation and incompleteness. Long writes:

> If there is no stable or foundational meaning, no one true sex, no one true religion, then the hermaphrodites are protean beings who change to suit their circumstances. Thus, not only are they of dual nature, they are beings who can infinitely multiply their roles. They are self-supplementing creatures who have refused to accept the basic premises that buttress French society, and thus are free to reinvent themselves constantly. (229)

Though the early modern hermaphrodite (intersex) is not the same as the performance/play of gendered roles I will examine in this chapter, the freedom of multiplication and fragmentation is of interest to larger discussions about premodern representations of gender. This chapter will consider both the opportunities and challenges of living in a world of simultaneous redefinition and strict prescription. Using the case study of seventeenth-century transvestite François-Timoléon, Abbé of Choisy, this chapter will explore moments of textual embodiment that stand in tension with the courtly code. Choisy's self-creation in *The Transvestite Memoirs* is grounded in partialities and fragments, and it troubles the courtly self-representation genre. It is my contention that the very textualization of the Abbé's experience is a liberating one in the writing of an alternative to the script. Stephanie Hilger notes (2020) that "sexually ambiguous bodies have occupied the human imagination since antiquity" (22). But she also goes on to specify that the eighteenth century is a period that "moved ambiguously sexed bodies from mythology to the scientific realm" (23). While the bodies I will be discussing here are not ambiguously sexed, they are ambiguously gendered, and there is a parallel interest in moving the body into the realm of control and erasing its ambiguity, even as central questions regarding the relationship between body and identity remain at stake. At the very moment when early modern elite culture is prescribing what it means to be a man, Choisy's counternarrative troubles expectations with a series of fragments, contradictions, and performances that give the reader the possibility to imagine a "trans" identity.

Courtly Handbooks and Self-representation

Before turning to Choisy's text, I will first briefly contextualize a few of the most relevant frameworks underlying performative self-representation in the courtly handbooks. Courtly men and women are driven to perpetuate fragmented (and often very gendered) images of themselves.

If the life of a courtier was codified into a written technology of behaviors, the practical application of these behaviors was a set of repetitive visual performances. A courtier's identity was both textually determined, by the prescriptive code of actions he sought to internalize, and visually determined, since his success was measured by the ability to reenact and perform his own version of the perfect courtier.[2] In Castiglione's text (2002), social networking spaces necessitate performances that are perfectly crafted and seemingly effortless. Ludovico outlines the goal:

[2] When referring to courtiers in general, I will use male pronouns, since most courtly handbooks were written for and by men. That is not to say that conduct manuals for women do not exist, and more work is beginning to be one on the role they played in courtly society. See, for example, Anne Larsen, "Marie Bruneau, Dame des Loges: Salon Conversation and the honnête femme. *Esprit Créateur*, Writing/Creating in the Feminine in Early Modern France, vol. 60, no. 1, 2020, pp. 100–112.

> to practice in all things a certain *sprezzatura*,[3] so as to conceal all art and make whatever is done or said appear to be without effort and almost without any thought about it … therefore we may call that art true which does not seem to be art; nor must one be more careful of anything than of concealing it, because if it is discovered, this robs a man of all credit and causes him to be held in slight esteem. (1.26.32)

The notion that the self is a series of inhabited roles, or performances, or masks, has been prolifically theorized and circulated in a variety of settings and disciplines. J.L.L. Austin's idea of performativity (1975), applied specifically to speech acts, suggests that the very utterance of a series of words creates their meaning; i.e., authenticity is established by performing the very words that one wishes to be true. For Judith Butler (1999), whose focus is the performativity of gender roles, performing a behavior or series of behaviors perpetuates the culturally determined roles that we come to identify as gendered. For Michel Foucault in *Discipline and Punish* (1977), individuals are accustomed to the idea of being constantly watched until they eventually perpetuate the surveillance internally (37). Surveillance becomes discursive. These frameworks continue to be relevant in the context of identity, and how people think of themselves in relationship to others, how they represent themselves to others, and how they watch themselves being watched. The notion of the self in the early modern period, and the relationship between this self and others, was in the very process of being shaped and defined.[4] Stephen Greenblatt's (2005) assertion in *Renaissance Self-Fashioning* that the early modern self is rhetorical, constructed out of layers of self-estrangement, started a decades-long debate about the nature and evolution of the self. In both the early modern period and today, there exists an uneasiness about how much of oneself to reveal. This very uneasiness inscribes individuals into a messy, dialogic, and self-perpetuating network of relationships.

[3] Most modern English translations use *nonchalance*; in keeping the original, I seek to invoke the complexity evoked by the Italian.

[4] One logical place to begin a discussion of the early modern self would be Michel de Montaigne's 1580 *Essays* (1958). In his introduction to the reader, Montaigne proclaims: "I am myself the matter of my book" (3), and he spends the better part of thirty years working on and revising that matter. In the seventeenth century, Cartesian dualisms and an increasing imperative to control the exterior passions are reflected in the codification of behavior and "self" that we see in courtly handbooks.

It is worth considering some of the potential consequences of living in a world that places such a heavy emphasis on *sprezzatura*. In the world of the early modern court, reputations could be built and—especially—lost in the moment of a slip or a failed performance. As a result, the stakes, and anxiety of self-representation, were high. As Wayne Rebhorn (1978) writes, "more important than the reflection [the courtier] sees in his mirror is the reflection of himself he sees in others' eyes (30). The performance of an individual was never individual but rather, inscribed into a *mise en abyme* of never-ending mirrors, performances and observations, resulting in a "culture of suspicion" (Berger Jr. 2002, 299). The discussion in the second book of Castiglione's text focuses on the pitfalls and apprehensiveness surrounding the agenda of the courtier. In the early modern world, each courtier must maximize his own chance to make a good impression, even—or in particular—at the cost of others. At the same time as he must make his own performance look easy, he must be constantly aware that others are watching him, looking for cracks in his performance.

The high stakes of this kind of negotiation are reflected in Nicholas Faret's *L'honneste homme, ou l'art de plaire à la court* (1630). Written a century after *The Book of the Courtier*, it is largely an adaptation of Castiglione's text for the French court. It eliminates the frame narrative and is straightforward in its presentation of ideal behaviors (and those to avoid) for members of elite society. Another key difference is the prevalence of passages that self-consciously paint the picture of the dangers involved in making a bad first impression. Faret warns readers that "before setting sail on a stormy ocean, it would be very useful to stand back for a bit and consider its condition. In this way, one will have the leisure to prepare, and to execute one's projects with prudence and dexterity" (Faret 1925, 38).[5] In other words, it is essential to "read the room," to consider court a dangerous place full of traps and secrets. In a culture where everyone is watching and everyone is suspicious, better to wait until one understands the rules of the game than to make a mistake and therefore ruin a first impression. Later on in the text, Faret concludes that it would be safest to "let us therefore be masters of ourselves, and know how to command our own affectations, if we wish to gain those of others" (Faret 69). Performances are meant to be planned carefully, executed perfectly, and crafted into one clear narrative.

[5] All translations from this text are mine.

The courtly handbook genre is primarily one that prescribes behaviors to male courtiers, but women play an implicit role in many of these texts. What qualities should the ideal lady possess? Should she be a complementary equal to the male courtier, or an imperfect version, in line with contemporary early modern discussions about women as anatomically imperfect versions of men? In *Making Sex*, Thomas Laqueur (1990) argues that such passages are "rampant with anxiety, expressed in the language of the body" (125). Castiglione's *Courtier* discursively rehearses and reinforces gender roles in many of its passages. Book three of the *Courtier*, in particular, contains lengthy discussions of differences between male and female courtiers, and their respective places in noble society. These passages emphasize classification and essentializing gender, moving away from ambiguity and gaps. Signor Magnifico notes that "a woman ought to be very unlike a man; for just as he must show a certain solid and sturdy manliness, so it is seemly for a woman to have a soft and delicate tenderness, with an air of womanly sweetness in her every movement, which, in her going and staying, and in whatever she says, shall always make her appear the woman without any resemblance to a man" (Castiglione 2002, 206).

Though they are filled with a certain kind of gender anxiety, to focus on these passages purely as straightforward manifestations of anxiety, as Laqueur does, is to ignore the deeper significance of *sprezzatura* and its relation to gender and performance. While discussing music, the Magnifico does label certain musical instruments unseemly for women. But he emphasizes that when a woman does make music or dance, she should "begin by letting herself be begged a little, and with a certain shyness bespeaking a noble shame that is the opposite of brazenness" (Castiglione 2002, 3.8.154). When comparing her own physical appearance and stature to other women, he continues, it is important to simultaneously be self-aware and pretend not to be: "if she is a little stouter or thinner than normal, or fair or dark, let her help herself in her dress, but in as hidden a way as possible; and all the while … let her appear to have no care or concern for this" (Castiglione 2002, 3.8.154). While there are clear ontological distinctions between the two sexes in Castiglione's reading, they share a very important quality: the ability to perform meaning using their bodies.[6] Women, like men, are meant to rehearse and perform a single narrative of self-representation using their bodies.

[6] See Katherine Crawford, *Perilous Performances: Gender and Regency in Early Modern France* (Harvard UP, 2004).

While it can create anxiety, *sprezzatura* also has the capacity to be used in the service of a different kind of self-representation, one that can disembody the self from the expectations of gender roles. If courtly handbooks establish the rules of the game, can effective use of *sprezzatura* dissolve those rules? How might gender distinctions that appear to divide men and women actually be used as subversive performative techniques? Choisy's narrative is by no means the only example of texts showing an interest in problematizing the binary gendered experience of the time. In *The Story of the Marquise-Marquis de Banneville* (Choisy et al. 2004), largely believed to be a collaboration between the Abbé de Choisy, Marie-Jeanne L'Héritier, and Charles Perrault, the two main characters are raised as the sex not assigned to them at birth: a boy is raised as a girl, as his mother fears that he will be drafted into war and killed like her late husband, and a girl who prefers to wear garments and always passes as male in public. In the end, the two fall in love, realize the truth about each other, but determine to go on living as they have been raised:

> "I am so accustomed to being a girl that I want to remain a woman all my life. How could I wear a man's hat?"
>
> "As for me," said the Marquis, "I have had my sword in my hand more than once without being ill at-ease, and I shall tell you my story one day. So let us remain as we are. Rejoice, beautiful Marquise, in all the charms of your sex, and I shall enjoy the freedom of mine." (129)

While the binary is reinforced at the end of the text—girl marries boy—the fluidity of gender remains open, since both characters feel most comfortable in their transitional identities. Turning now to the case study of the Abbé de Choisy invites us to "reflect on the meanings of men traversing gender boundaries" (Seifert 2009, 207) and to consider the role of *sprezzatura* in disrupting and rewriting gendered self-representation in the early modern period.

Case Study: François-Timoléon, Abbé de Choisy (1644–1724)

Raised at the court of Louis XIV, François-Timélon, Abbé de Choisy was surrounded by courtiers and *sprezzatura* from childhood. Jeanne Olympe raised her fourth son as a girl, perhaps, some speculate, because after giving birth to three sons she wished, with her last child, already miraculously conceived when she was in her forties, to have a daughter. Patricia Cholakian (2000) has suggested that Jeanne "engineered [her son's] gender identity for political reasons" to curry the favor of Louis XIV by mirroring and thus normalizing his own brother's extra-normative cross-dressing" (155). Despite the fact that Louis XIV's brother openly cross-dressed, it should be noted that French law punished transvestism with death by fire until 1760.[7] Thus it is rather remarkable not only that the Abbé de Choisy was able to pull off a double life, and to document it so freely, but also that Choisy was elected to the Académie Française in 1687, taking a place alongside some of the giants of French Classicism such as Racine and Boileau (Greenberg 2001, 123).

In *The Transvestite Memoirs*, Choisy describes several episodes (roughly encompassing the decade of Choisy's twenties) during which they dress and are accepted as a beautiful woman.[8] In the first part of the text, people in Choisy's social circle are aware of their biological status as a man, but/and come to accept their self-presentation as a woman. In later parts of the text, the transvestism is not known, and Choisy successfully passes for a woman. Choisy repeatedly refers to their transvestism as "my old weaknesses" (28); at the same time, there are moments when Choisy expresses correspondence between their outward presentation as woman and their inner sense of self: "I had a gown of white damask lined with black taffeta, the train half an elle long … I felt truly a woman" (31). At the end of the *Memoirs*, the Abbé notes that while they decided to "give up … such trifling," they felt remorseful about it later in life, after having lost great sums of money to gambling: "I would have been happier if I had always made myself up as a beauty, even when I was ugly! Ridicule is preferable to poverty" (Choisy 1994, 102). The *Memoirs* are a collection of fragments and the motivation for their publication is unknown. What I wish to focus on here is the way in

[7] For a history of transvestism in early modern France, see Sylvie Steinberg, Sylvie, *La Confusion des sexes: le travestissement de la Renaissance à la Révolution* (Fayard, 2001). For an excellent study of gender and queer culture in early modern France, see Gary Ferguson, *Queer (Re)Readings in the French Renaissance: Homosexuality, Gender, Culture* (Ashgate, 2008). For an account that focuses specifically on cross dressing, see Joseph Harries, *Hidden Agendas: Cross-Dressing in 17th Century France* (Gunter Narr Verlag, 2005).

[8] Except where noted, I have decided to use non-binary pronouns for Choisy. It is true that Choisy decides to return to exclusively living and dressing as a man at the end of the *Memoirs*. But my choice of pronoun reflects the non-binary experience that the text gives us, even if it is deeply problematic at times.

which Choisy uses text—the medium of prescriptive, gender-enforcing courtly handbooks—as a tool of self-presentation in which Choisy engages.

In an early passage, Choisy begins attending balls and other public performances in drag, and enjoys not being recognized: "When I was at a ball or the theatre, wearing my beautiful *robes de chambre*, diamonds and patches, and heard people murmur near me 'There is a lovely woman', I experienced an inward glow of pleasure which is incomparable" (Choisy 1994, 30). Choisy is aware of being looked at, and enjoys the validation and success of their carefully-crafted performance. They go on to write, "it is sweet to deceive the eyes of the public" (86). It would appear that Choisy thrives in an environment where visual performance allows for the perpetuation of an ideal. But herein lies one of the interpretive challenges of Choisy's memoir. It is never clear to readers when, or if, or to what extent, the narrator is being authentic.[9] As Mitchell Greenberg writes (2001), it is difficult to "fix Choisy into a discursive narration … by whatever criterion we try to approach him, he escapes our grasp" (124). This unsettling of certainty is what separates Choisy from the normative genre of courtly writing, but it also makes it very difficult to know how to interpret the various versions of Choisy that readers encounter in the text.

Abbé de Choisy goes to great lengths in order to pull off a performance, and the text itself is very performative. Many passages spend paragraphs at a time describing the dress, the hair style, and the accessories involved in each evening's appearance. Almost universally, Choisy notes (1994) that "no one could have guessed that I was not a woman" (71). There are some exceptions that indicate to readers that the anxieties and prescriptions of acceptable gender performance were present in Choisy's life. At one cultural excursion, Monsieur de Montausier approaches Choisy and confronts them, proclaiming, "I admit, madame, or mademoiselle, I do not know what to call you, I admit that you are beautiful, but have you no shame at wearing such clothing and acting as a woman, seeing that you are fortunate enough not to be one? Go, go and hide yourself!" (65). Choisy shows no reaction to this particular moment or to other occasional exceptions to their universal acclaim as a celebrated beauty, but there are moments where readers get a sense that Choisy is ashamed of non-conformity and their subversive performances. It is evident that they go to great lengths to avoid being negatively

[9] See Paul Scott (2015), who posits that Choisy's memoirs are completely fictional. Though we cannot include discussion of Scott's work her for reasons of space, it surely adds new perspective to the conversation.

talked about; for example, "[o]ne day, I risked going to the Comédie with my dear Maulny and her aunt, but I was stared at too much, I was too much the object of attention … it was a long time before I returned there; I had to avoid scandal" (43).

It is important to take seriously the argument that Choisy (1994) constructs an artificial identity in order to manipulate and take sexual advantage of young girls. Having brought on a fifteen year-old girl named Babet as his personal maid, the young girl goes to bed with Choisy, thinking that he is a woman. There, "I kissed her three or four times most enjoyably. I put her, all of her, between my legs and greatly fondled her" (50). This sort of scenario is repeated often and textually recounted in great detail (86), with the author always taking pleasure in the trick of the gender performance and the sexual pleasure that he experiences.[10]

Regardless of Choisy's motivations, it is clear that their text is part of the performance. The self-stated need to be seen (evidenced by Choisy's theatrical performances of sex acts in front of others) is mimetically repeated by textually reproducing each performance to readers and by creating a kind of double mirror. In the *Memoirs*, Choisy's text stands in for their body. It reflects the same kind of multiplicity that defines who "Choisy" is. One could conclude that Choisy inhabits a "transitional subjectivity" (Seifert 2009, 227), representing an early modern experience that might be considered one of the "forerunners of transgendered existence" and linking gender to personhood (Seifert 2009, 211–12). Even as Seifert argues for Choisy's transitional experience, he also concedes that Choisy does not fit into any of the available categories that preceded the term 'transgender' (213). Choisy is intentionally and repeatedly disconnected from categories in a system defined by obsessive categorization. I believe that the most authentic moments in Choisy's sometimes subversive use of the courtly vocabulary are those in which they are most fragmented, in the moments when readers are asked to fill in the gaps between irony, performance, and authenticity—in the "unresolved tension" that defines much of Choisy's life (Seifert 2009, 232).

One thing that is clear from the outset is the extent to which Choisy is extremely self-aware within their own text; indeed, textual self-awareness is itself part of the narrative and part of the body that Choisy presents to readers. The text reflects the tensions and fragmentation, the multiplicities

[10] I am using male pronouns in this paragraph to reflect the unambiguous exploitation that takes place during Choisy's sexual encounters with young girls.

that define its author. Without the words of the memoir, readers would not have access to Choisy's cross-dressed body. This makes the text—in its fragmented, and at times contradictory form—an undeniable part of Choisy's body language. The text is as necessary to their image as the earrings, patches and flourishes with which they adorn themself. During one encounter with Madame de Lafayette, celebrated writer and member of the intellectual elite, Choisy notes that the former "me as a good friend that this was not right for a man, and I would do better by far to dress myself totally as a woman" (62–63). The reference to another writer—and not just any writer, but one whose own texts pay great attention to outward appearances and performances—validates Choisy's body within the textual realm and posits the performance of gender as a textual collaboration between Lafayette and Choisy.

Even years later, Choisy takes pride in re-scripting and re-viewing himself in his own words. As Greenberg (2001) writes, Choisy works to create their identity "not in the reality of the body … but in its displacement, in the symbolic exchanges of the sexed body into and as the material construction of a body image" (319–40). This takes place gradually, fluidly, and not always linearly: "So, by degrees, I accustomed people to seeing me dressed up in this way" (Choisy 1994, 29). The process of "becoming" is replicated in the repeated textual fragmentation, as readers, too, become accustomed to seeing Choisy as a woman. This is a queer renegotiation of the *Courtier*: On one hand, Choisy embodies exactly the kind of courtier that Castiglione had in mind. Their *sprezzatura* is one of mirrors, twists, and dazzling rhetoric. But it is also one of uneasiness and instability. Readers are never sure just what kind of performance to expect. Choisy's performance shows that *sprezzatura* can be successfully used to embody a queer self, and to call that queerness into question: Choisy's masks, made from makeup and clothing, function as both shields and weapons.

Choisy's embodiment is realized in the paragraphs of the *Memoirs*; their story is textually created. At the same time, the text *re*creates their body. Readers have access to elements of Choisy's performances that characters in the story explicitly and deliberately do not. "No one could have guessed that I was not a woman," writes Choisy (71). After so many fragmented performances, so much work to "[shape and condition]," so many "processes of transition" (Ferguson 2013, 151), readers are left with the question: "who *is* Choisy"? It is unclear whether or not the author of the memoirs knows the answer. But *sprezzatura*, set into motion by handbooks such as Castiglione's and perfected at the court of Louis XIV, gives

Choisy the textual and performative vocabulary to fluidly explore this question. They are able to embody *sprezzatura* in a way that brings to life one of the presumptive goals of the courtly handbooks: to perform a role until you *embody* the very identity that you wish to inhabit. But the instability of Choisy's embodiment, and the re-textualization of this very performance, renegotiates the very definition of *sprezzatura*. To perform and to write, for Choisy, is a visual and textual tool that renegotiates the definition of *sprezzatura*: rather than reinforce the gender norms of the time, Choisy's queer *sprezzatura* transforms the gendered experience into something that can also be liberating. This stands in explicit contrast to other queer bodies at court. The King's brother Philippe de France, known as *Monsieur*, whose effeminate nature and preference for male lovers was publicly known, is described as being envious of Choisy's freedom: "I went to the Palais-Royal whenever Monsieur was in Paris. He was almost effusively friendly to me, because we had the same inclinations. He longed to dress as a woman himself, but did not dare, because of his position (princes are prisoners of their rank)" (1994, 63). Choisy accomplishes reinvention by turning upside down the very mechanism that resists deviation from the norm—the courtly handbook, which defines and (here) imprisons the elite of high rank. Choisy uses the prescriptive genre of extreme exteriority in order to un-prescribe, redefine, and destabilize what it means to perform gender in the seventeenth century. Visual cues, performative presentations, and the subversion of any boundaries between male and female—fluidly, sometimes violently, moving between both—the Abbé de Choisy leaves readers to fill in the gaps and to decide what, about their gendered performances, is real.

Later in the seventeenth century, a new generation of handbooks, rejecting the premise of the *Courtier*, suggest that the ideal courtier should strive for something more authentic, drawing his identity from "the inner space of the self" (Seifert 2009, n24). For example, Antoine de Courtin (1672) writes that the goal of a courtier is to "aspirer à quelque chose de plus solide" than a convincing performance. But how can one achieve "authenticity" when that very concept is created out of other performances, other codifications, and other words? It would be easy to conclude that the success of a courtier is perpetuated by a performative shell consisting of the echoes of other words. Surely, courtiers doing their best to succeed in an environment of extreme exteriority would be aware that "what appears is seldom the truth" (Lafayette 1678 (1994), 19). As I have argued elsewhere, courtly handbooks both create and are created by the extreme exteriority of the courtly world (Peterson 2016, 98). And yet this same extreme exteriority that seeks to stabilize and categorize what it means to be a man can also, in its fragmentation, trouble these very categories and add fluidity to our understanding of the gender experience of the late seventeenth century.

Bibliography

Austin, J.L.L. *How to Do Things With Words*, Harvard UP, 1975.

Berger Jr., Harry. "Sprezzatura and the Absence of Grace." In *The Book of the Courtier*, edited by Daniel Javitch, Norton, 2002, pp. 295–307.

Butler, Judith. *Gender Trouble: Feminism and the Subversion of Identity*, Routledge, 1999.

Castiglione, Baldassare. *The Book of the Courtier*, 1528. Translated by Charles Singleton, edited by Daniel Javitch, Norton, 2002, pp. 1–260.

Choisy, François Timoléon, Abbé de. *The Transvestite Memoirs and the Story of the Marquise Marquis de Banneville*. Translated, with an introduction by R.H.F. Scott. Peter Owen, 1994, pp. 27–102.

Choisy, Françoise-Timoléon, Abbé de, Marie-Jeanne L'Héritier, and Charles Perrault. *The Story of the Marquise-Marquis de Banneville*. Translated by Steven Rendall, Introduction and notes by Joan DeJean, MLA Texts & Translations, 2004.

Cholakian, Patricia. *Women and the Politics of Self-Representation in Seventeenth Century France*, U of Delaware P, 2000.

Courtin, Antoine de. *Nouveau Traité de la Civilité qui se pratique en France, parmi les honnestes Gens*, Paris, Helie Josset, 2nd ed., 1672.

Crawford, Katherine, *Perilous Performances: Gender and Regency in Early Modern France*, Harvard UP, 2004.

Faret, Nicolas. *L'honneste homme ou: l'art de plaire à la court*. 1636. Ed. M. Magendie. PUF, 1925.

Ferguson, Gary. "Early Modern Transitions: From Montaigne to Choisy." *L'Esprit Créateur*, vol. 53, no. 1, Transgender France, Spring 2013, pp. 145–157.

Ferguson, Gary. *Queer (Re)Readings in the French Renaissance: Homosexuality, Gender, Culture*, Ashgate, 2008.

Foucault, Michel. *Discipline and Punish: The Birth of the Prison*. Translated by Alan Sheridan, Vintage Books, 1977.

Goffman, Erving. *The Presentation of the Self in Everyday Life*, University of Edinburgh Social Sciences Research Centre, 1956.

Greenberg, Mitchell. *Baroque Bodies: Psychoanalysis and the Culture of French Absolutism*, Cornell UP, 2001.

Greenblatt, Stephen. *Renaissance Self-Fashioning: From More to Shakespeare*, University of Chicago Press, 2nd ed., 2005.

Harries, Joseph, *Hidden Agendas: Cross-Dressing in 17th Century France*. Tübingen, Gunter Narr Verlag, 2005.

Hilger, Stephanie. "Epistemological Anxiety: The Case of Michel-Anne Drouart." *Bodies in Transition in the Health Humanities*, edited by Lisa M. DeTora and Stephanie Hilger, Routledge, 2020, pp. 22–34.

Lafayette, Marie-Madeleine de. *The Princesse of Clèves*. Edited and translated by John D. Lyons, Norton, 1994.

Laqueur, Thomas, *Making Sex: Body and Gender from the Greeks to Freud*, Harvard UP, 1990.

Larsen, Anne. "Marie Bruneau, Dame des Loges: Salon Conversation and the honnête femme. *Esprit Créateur*, Writing/Creating in the Feminine in Early Modern France, vol. 60, no. 1, 2020, pp. 100–112.

Long, Kathleen P., *Hermaphrodites in Renaissance Europe*, Ashgate, 2006.

Montaigne, Michel de. *The Complete Essays of Montaigne*, translated by Donald M. Frame, Stanford UP, 1958.

Peterson, Nora Martin. *Involuntary Confessions of the Flesh in Early Modern France*, U of Delaware P, 2016.

Rebhorn, Wayne. *Courtly Performances: Masking and Festivity in Casiglione's* Book of the Courtier, Wayne State UP, 1978.

Scott, Paul. "Authenticity and Textual Transvestism in the Memoirs of Abbé de Choisy." French Studies, vol. 69, no. 1 (2015): pp. 14–29.

Seifert, Lewis. *Manning the Margins: Masculinity and Writing in Seventeenth Century France*, U of Michigan P, 2009.

Steinberg, Sylvie, *La Confusion des sexes: le travestissement de la Renaissance à la Révolution*, Fayard, 2001.

Stryker, Susan. "(De)Subjugated Knowledges: An Introduction to Transgender Studies." In *The Transgender Studies Reader*, edited by Susan Stryker and Stephen Whittle, Routledge, 2006, 1–17.

Theaters of Psychosomatics

Sophie Witt

Introduction[1]

A famous image from the history of medicine—André Brouillet's *Une Leçon Clinique à la Salpêtrière*, painted in 1887—shows the neurologist Jean-Martin Charcot during one of his famous *Leçons du Mardi* (Tuesday lessons).[2] A fascinated male audience views a hypnotized female "hysteric," Blanche Wittmann. Art historian Georges Didi-Huberman (2003) described Charcot's clinic as *théâtre* (theater):

> A reciprocity of charm was instituted between physicians, with their insatiable desire for images of Hysteria, and hysterics, who willingly participated

[1] The article forms part of the project, "The Medical Knowledge of Theater: History of Fascination and Poetics of Psychosomatics (1750–1970)" at the University of Zurich. For more information see: https://www.ds.uzh.ch/de/projekte/psychosomatik.html.

[2] https://commons.wikimedia.org/wiki/File:Une_leçon_clinique_à_la_Salpêtrière.jpg. Brouillet, André. "Une leçon clinique à la Salpêtrière (1887)," Museé d'histoire de la médicine, Paris, cited in Didi-Huberman (2003), 238.

S. Witt (✉)
University of Hamburg, Hamburg, Germany
e-mail: sophie.witt@uni-hamburg.de

J. Cressman et al. (eds.), *Envisioning Embodiment in the Health Humanities*, Sustainable Development Goals Series,
https://doi.org/10.1007/978-3-031-49807-7_3

> and actually raised the stakes through their increasingly theatricalized bodies. In this way, hysteria in the clinic became the spectacle, the *invention of hysteria*. Indeed, hysteria was covertly identified with something like an art, close to theater or painting. (xi)

Some 50 years later, Helen Flanders Dunbar, founder of US-American psychosomatics, publishes *Mind and Body: Psychosomatic Medicine* (1947; c.f. Powell 1977). The introduction to the second edition states that "knowledge has been acquired which permits more positive statements about the concomitants of emotional and physical disorders. Much has been learned about 'ailments' which a few years ago were labeled 'cause unknown'" (Dunbar 1966, 1). Despite this confident tone, Dunbar provides not scientific explanations but rather melodramatic "case histories" and full-blown bourgeois tragedies enacted among mothers, fathers, children. This connection to theatricality is foreshadowed by an epigrammatic quotation from Shakespeare's *King Lear*: "We are not ourselves / When nature, being oppress'd, commands the mind / To suffer with the body" (II.4.103–07).[3] Dunbar's connection of the theater and psychosomatics is not incidental.

I argue that a study of the history of psychosomatics must include a humanities perspective that centers on the specific and "disruptive" mediality of theatricality, that is, the combination of verbal speech, bodily signs, and aspects of space and timing.[4] I propose that the function of theatrical metaphors or figures of thought is dual: first, to make *visible* the *invisible* psychic dimensions of illnesses, by means of staging and observing the body in a specific environment (*Umwelt*) and situatedness; and second, to reflect on the epistemologically problematic—always only *partial*—character of this hermeneutical endeavor.[5]

[3] Quoted in Dunbar (1966), 1.

[4] For a critical review of the pivotal role of narrativity in medical humanities and a plea for "post-narrative," see Woods (2011a, 2011b, 2012) and Whitehead and Woods (2016). The most popular and highly cited text within the corpus of medical humanities' reliance on narrative is Frank (1995).

[5] For an epistemology of the partial, see Haraway (1991).

Psychosomatics Between Biomedical Explanations and Hermeneutics

Charcot's clinic is a "primal scene" in the history of psychosomatics: Sigmund Freud's interest in hysteria originated from his visit to the Salpêtrière. In *Studies on Hysteria* (1895), Freud (1955) and Breuer "discover," rather unintentionally, so-called conversion, i.e., "the transformation of psychical excitation into chronic somatic symptoms" (122) as the core "hysterical method of defence" (86). Although the psychoanalytic foundation of psychosomatic theory later was questioned (for example in the case of Georg Groddeck's psychoanalytical symbolism) the idea of conversion endured, notably in Thure von Uexküll's influential formulation. Psychosomatics is based on a "[t]ransformation of mental contents into physical symptoms" (Uexküll, 1963, 82) (he notes, staying thus with the concept of "hysterical trouble."

Since the days of the Salpêtrière, theatricality has not been limited to the visible staging of hysterical symptoms. Rather, theatricality suffuses the clinical scene, which creates an epistemological dilemma. It is precisely by bringing the symptom to an observable surface that its evident truth-status and objective explicability vanish: "Hypnotic theater, insofar as it is 'mastered' by the 'fascinator,' *demarcates and intensifies the symptom*: it constrains the symptom to the perfection of a drawing, which, in its *artifice*, provides something like the truth of the symptomatic event in itself" (Didi-Huberman, 2003, 244). In other words, the price of making the symptom visible is its inseparability from the frame in which it is staged for observation—in relation to which it is only *readable*.

What might appear limited to the "era of hypnosis" and its shady methods has lingered on as an epistemological and semiotic question. Uexküll observes that psychosomatics should be approached from the perspective of the relationship between verbal and embodied processes of signification. A psychosomatic symptom represents an inherent failure of universal signification. The "psychosomatic observer [...] leaves the standpoint of 'spectator from outside' and the realm of ethological physiology ... [and] starts creating hypotheses about something that occurs inside the observed system .... This means he insinuates that the stimulus is a sign carrier that has a specific meaning within the semantic boundaries of the living system under observation" (Uexküll, 1982, 209). In other words, psychosomatics *contests* any form of un-situated knowledge claims, in this case, biomedicine's notion of illness as a "disturbance of a [...] physico-biochemical machine" (Uexküll, 1982, 206) and of symptoms "as events of an objective world" (Uexküll, 1982, 211).

Problems of (in-)explicability and the intertwinement of medical knowledge with hermeneutical procedures also informed the most recent update to the *Diagnostic and Statistical Manual of Mental Disorders* (DSM5), of the American Psychiatric Association (American Psychiatric Association, 2013). DSM5 collects phenomena of "conversion"—i.e., medically inexplicable "transformations" from the psychic into the somatic register—under the umbrella term "Somatic Symptom Disorder and related disorders." The DSM essentially reconceptualized existing "somatization disorders," "somatoform disorders," "pain disorders," "hypochondriasis," or "factitious disorders," among others. The authors described these "sweeping changes" especially with respect to the "conversive" somatoform disorders (since DSM-III), whose "defining characteristic was the concept of 'Medically Unexplained Symptoms'" (Dimsdale et al., 2013, 223). In contrast, DSM5 defines the disorder on the basis of persistent somatic symptoms associated with disproportionate thoughts, feelings, and behaviors related to these symptoms" (Dimsdale et al., 2013, 223). This "major change" produced much discussion and critique, including a warning of the potential "risk" of "mislabeling many as mentally ill" (Frances, 2013, 26).

What interests me here is the translation of criteria of medical (in-) explicability into the very different paradigm of semiotics and hermeneutics. Whereas DSM-III and -IV focused on the potential biomedical causes of symptoms, the "thoughts, feelings, and behaviors" discussed in the new DSM-V emphasize processes of *interpretation*: What are the respective thoughts, feelings, and behaviors in each and every individual case? To what extent are they "disproportional?" And as compared with which "normal" emotional or mental condition of this or that person? Interpretation strongly depends on the (quasi-scenic) standpoint of the interpreter along with their relation to what is observed. Both observer and observed are part of a specific spatiotemporal situatedness. Importantly, the United States is alone in seeing psychosomatic medicine primarily as a subspecialty of psychiatry and neurology.[6] In Germany and many other European countries, psychosomatics has widely been considered a subspecialty of internal medicine, and from the 1970s onward has even been

[6] For psychiatry's struggle to explain mental disorder in biomedical terms cf. Harrington (2019).

regarded as a core attitude of clinicians *in general*. A German textbook on psychosomatics and psychotherapy notes that "around one third of illnesses are caused by psychological or psychosocial factors," and that beyond the question of diagnosis and treatment of specific illnesses, psychosomatics would point toward a psychological or psychosocial understanding of clinical medicine in general by claiming a bio-psycho-social orientation toward all questions of illness and health (Ermann et al., 2009, 9ff., translation mine).

I thus propose that psychosomatic illnesses should be included in a critical discussion of the "widening of the sites and scales of 'the medical,'" in the sense that William Viney, Felicity Callard, and Angela Woods suggest (Viney et al., 2015, 2). Since psychosomatics attests to the *limits* of biomedicine and its scientific methods of explanation, new vocabulary and imagery are needed to comprehend and imagine the rather uncanny relation between soma and psyche, body and signs, nature and culture (c.f. Mitscherlich 2010). A bio-psycho-social orientation means, at least theoretically, that one *reads* illnesses and its bodily symptoms as *signs for something else*, as semiotic and communicative phenomena, as culturally specific and historically dependent experiences and concepts. Psychosomatics thus shifts "the medical" from the realm of the natural sciences—and from the scene of the clinical encounter—into the cultural sphere and perhaps even literary studies, in that it introduces (biographical) semiotics and hermeneutics to scientific explanations. This aligns with ideas espoused in the "Critical Medical Humanities," which call for "recognition that the arts, humanities and social sciences are best viewed not as in service or in opposition to the clinical and life sciences, but as productively entangled with a 'biomedical culture' [...]" (Viney et al., 2015, 2).[7] Psychosomatics, in this view, can *only* be understood transdisciplinarily, at the intersection of medical/natural science and humanities. But considering that there is no psychosomatics without the arts and the humanities, its history also appears to be much older and broader than that of its fledgling existence as medi-

[7] In "Entangling the Medical Humanities" Fitzgerald & Callard (2016) argue against "a model of *integration*" of the humanities, and thus against the first important wave of medical humanities in the UK context that has been concerned with training medical practitioners, namely by integrating concepts and methods of the humanities and social sciences into the medical curricula. During the past years, a second wave of "critical" medical humanities called for an extension of these areas of work and for more theoretically based approaches, based on critical theory and poststructuralist thought. *Critical* medical humanities are comparable to the field of Health Humanities in the US context. See also Macneill (2011).

cal discipline.[8] One of the intriguing examples from the eighteenth century is Friedrich Schiller, studied physician and writer, especially playwright (1781a, 1781b). The next chapter deals with his ideas of psychosomatics before I return to the theoretical discussion of the role of theatricality within Critical Medical Humanities.

Psychophysical Drama and "No Trace of Wound"

Friedrich Schiller's debut play, *The Robbers. A Tragedy* (1781a) depicts sibling rivalry exacerbated by the conflict between the least favorite son, Francis, and his father Maximilian, Count von Moor. The drama leads inexorably to Francis's attempt to kill his father. While this is a rather classic tragic—and Oedipal—conflict and storyline, it is in Schiller's work not confined merely to the realm of the psychological. Rather, from the opening lines, it is the infirmity of the *biological body* through which the psychological conflict is made *visible* in a very literal manner: Father Moor is "pale" and is stated as having a "feeble frame" ("einen zerbrechlichen Körper") while being still healthy enough to wonder with suspicion about his son's "anxiety about [the father's] health" (Schiller, 1781a/2014, Act I/Scene 1). Moreover it is precisely this medical notion of the body's infirmity that prompts Francis's thinking when he decides to try to kill his father. This is the plan:

> FRANCIS. I should like to do what your clever physician does, only the reverse way—not stop Nature's course by running a bar across her path, but only help her to speed a little faster. Are we not able to prolong the conditions of life? Why, then, should we not also be able to shorten them? Philosophers and physiologists teach us how close is the sympathy between the emotions of the mind and the movements of the bodily machine. Convulsive sensations are always accompanied by a disturbance of the mechanical vibrations—passions injure the vital powers—an overburdened spirit bursts its shell. Well, then—what if one knew how to smooth this unbeaten path, for the easier entrance of death into the citadel of life?—to work the body's destruction through the mind—ha! an original device!—who can accomplish this?—a device without a parallel! (Act II/Scene I)

[8] Psychosomatics is brought into focus of clinical medicine systematically only from the 1920s onward – first in Europe, later on in the US. For the German-speaking context, see the recent volume edited by Geisthövel & Hitzer (2019).

Departing from the common idea of a close relation between mind and body in late eighteenth-century German *Anthropologie*,[9] Francis obsesses over destructive psychic effects ("to work the body's destruction through the mind"). In what follows, he ponders over the potential fatal impact of specific "species of sensation": "And how, then, must I, too, go to work to dissever that sweet and peaceful union of soul and body?" Francis thus reverses the idea, popular in the eighteenth century, that a healthy mind resides in a healthy body, and vice versa. And so he continues:

> Anger?—that ravenous wolf is too quickly satiated. Care? that worm gnaws far too slowly. Grief?—that viper creeps too lazily for me. Fear?—hope destroys its power. What! and are these the only executioners of man? is the armory of death so soon exhausted? (In deep thought.) How now! what! ho! I have it! (Starting up.) Terror! What is proof against terror? What powers have religion and reason under that giant's icy grasp! And yet—if he should withstand even this assault? If he should! Oh, then, come Anguish to my aid! and thou, gnawing Repentance!—furies of hell, burrowing snakes who regorge your food, and feed upon your own excrements; ye that are forever destroying, and forever reproducing your poison! And thou, howling Remorse, that desolatest thine own habitation, and feedest upon thy mother. And come ye, too, gentle Graces, to my aid; even you, sweet smiling Memory, goddess of the past—and thou, with thy overflowing horn of plenty, blooming Futurity; show him in your mirror the joys of Paradise, while with fleeting foot you elude his eager grasp. Thus will I work my battery of death, stroke after stroke, upon his fragile body, until the troop of furies close upon him with Despair! Triumph! triumph! (Act II/Scene I)

Francis "meditates" over psychophysical correlations in their most pure and simple way. Parting from the "union of mind and body" the drama supposes a kind of coupling between the different levels of the mental and the bodily. But contrary to the eighteenth century's obsession with holism's *harmonizing* impact, Francis' monologue interestingly celebrates the "ugly feelings" as part of a potential "death drive," that will later be theorized by Freud. In Freud, the life drive is related to preservation, but also to *union*, while the death drive stands in for destructiveness and the

[9] See exemplarily Platner (1772); for 18th century holism, refer to Schings (1994).

dissolving of coherence.[10] Francis's "ugly," deadly feelings might thus be a "death trap" for theorizing psychophysical correlations as an unproblematic union and/or simple transference or translation. Correspondingly, the triumphant killing of the father does not work out in the drama very well: in Act V Old Moor finally indeed "expires" (in the German text he meaningfully "*gibt seinen Geist auf*," his plea for mental endurance—"keep my soul from sinking"—being obviously ignored). But at that moment, the would-be triumphant Francis is also already dead; far from mastering the sensation, he "strangles himself" in a state of psychic terror when the "troop of furies" finally comes after him: "Betrayed! betrayed! The spirit [sic] of the dead are vomited from their graves. The realm of death, shaken out of its eternal slumber, roars at me, 'Murderer, murderer!' Who moves there?" (Act V/Scene I).

Against this backdrop, it is interesting the way that Francis's extensive "meditation" on mind-body union proceeds: "Triumph! triumph!—the plan is complete—difficult and masterly beyond compare—sure—safe; for then (with a sneer) the dissecting knife can find *no trace of wound* or of corrosive poison" (Act II/Scene I; emphasis added). At first glance, the "dissecting knife" of forensics appears to suggest "triumph" on the side of a mechanistic worldview that considers "body as machine." However, the supposed forensic evidence is characterized as *categorically impossible*. A suffering or dead body with "no trace of wound" might not only point to "mental trauma" as a possible cause for ill health but can also be understood as paradigmatic figure of the "trauma" of examination and diagnosis. Not only does scientific explanation fail, but any possible sign of a semiotic order is either non-existent or at least unreadable. From this perspective, no evident or holistic knowledge emerges when we put "[p]hilosophers and physiologists" together, which was the universalist hope of German late seventeenth-century anthropology, on which early twentieth-century German psychosomatics relied.[11] If psychosomatics points to the interconnectedness of multiple categories in the sciences and humanities, a persistent uncertainty and uncanniness of the "missing trace" radically destabilizes all notions of both anthropological and epistemological

[10] For scholarly commentary on "death-drives," see Laplanche & Pontalis (2011), 502, (1974), p. 97ff. See also Freud (1941, p. 71):" "Nach langem Zögern und Schwanken haben wir uns entschlossen, nur zwei Grundtriebe anzunehmen, den *Eros* und den *Destruktionstrieb*. [...] Das Ziel des ersten ist, immer grössere Einheiten herzustellen und so zu erhalten, also Bindung, das Ziel des anderen im Gegenteil, Zusammenhänge aufzulösen und so die Dinge zu zerstören. Beim Destruktionstrieb können wir daran denken, dass als sein letztes Ziel erscheint, das Lebende in den anorganischen Zustand zu überführen. Wir heissen ihn darum auch *Todestrieb*."

[11] For this genealogy, see Harrington (2008). See exemplarily von Weizsäcker (1987).

holism. I thus agree with Monica Greco, who draws on Michel Foucault in her argument that we should approach psychosomatics "as a form of *problematization*" (Greco, 1998, 4):

> [T]he word "psychosomatic" does not refer to a specific content nor to a specific method [...]. Rather, "psychosomatics" is approached as what defines a space, a multiple and contradictory space, where something new is introduced as an object for thought. It is a space that includes the discursive and non-discursive practices that emerge when a domain of action or behaviour, illness in this case, has lost its customary familiarity and has become uncertain, as a result of social, economic, or political processes. Here the primary connotation of the word "psychosomatic" is its contentiousness, its ambivalence, its availability for a definite variety of constructions and appropriations, which amount to its *problematic* character.[12]

A Case for Theatricality in Critical Medical Humanities

I will now link this notion of "lost familiarity" and "uncertainty" more concretely to the question of theatricality. One entry point into the topic is the use of theatrical metaphors in medical texts. Without delving too deeply into theories of metaphor, the close relationship between the functioning of a metaphor and the notion of visualization dates back at least to Aristotle's *energeia*, i.e., visualization.[13] Accordingly, metaphors seem to appear in these textbooks precisely because unfamiliar topics need to be visualized to the students. The *Textbook of Psychosomatic Medicine*, for instance, notes that the temptation to react in an "angry way" to "deceptive patients" would "only play into the patient's pathology by drawing the physician into a *dramatized scene*" (Levenson, 2011, 295; emphasis added). In this example, the "dramatized scene" is clearly connected to the patient's "pathological behavior" and their tendency to "self-fabricate," "simulate," "invent," or "exaggerate" somatic symptoms—in any case, "dramatized scene[s]" must be *avoided* by crafty psychiatrists. This anti-theatrical tone ties in with the psychiatrist's concern with "explanations" (Levenson, 2011, 298).

Yet, in other contexts, "scenes" and "staging" are labeled as *useful* "irrational" phenomena of doctor-patient-relations, as in a German textbook that explains "that in an interview much more is happening than the

[12] Greco makes reference to Foucault (1988). See also Foucault (1984).
[13] See Aristotle (1996).

exchange of objective data," and that students will learn to "discover and decrypt a 'scene,'" in this case, referring to the hidden psychic meanings revealed in the interaction of doctor and patient (Ermann et al. 15; translation mine). Although not objective, and therefore irritating and unfamiliar, "stagings" and "scenes" as part of the (counter-) transference processes within therapy are considered to be important tools and even seem to be the *only* way to gain access to the psychic dimensions of illness. There is an obvious *didactic* aim of metaphorical language in these two examples: (1) teaching future doctors their respective roles and (2) teaching the Health Humanities scholar that these roles differ tremendously with respect to the various notions of mental illness, diagnosis, and treatment. Even so, this acknowledgment of the "problematic," the "unfamiliar" or even "unknown" continues to be closely connected to theater as a figure of thought if we dig deeper into the medical theory of psychosomatics in the twentieth century.

Joyce McDougall posits her book *Theaters of the Body. A Psychoanalytical Approach to Psychosomatic Illness* (McDougall, 1989) as a counterforce to a hunt for semiotic expression. McDougall is one of the few analysts to have placed questions of theatricality explicitly at the center of her thinking. As she notes in her introduction, her theatrical thinking about psychosomatic illness originated from an irritation she experienced while working on *Theater of the Mind* (McDougall, 1991). In that book, she utilizes the metaphor of theater to shed light on the centrality of tragic conflict to the understanding of the economic and dynamic aspects of the 'I' whose aim is to "maintain meaning and to channel the forces of cathexis," as Weber states (Weber, 2000, 31). He points out that in McDougall's *Theatre of the Mind*, "the I [...] emerges [...] as star of the show: its hero and director at once" (31).

In *Theaters of the Body* (McDougall, 1989) the focus on tragic conflict and on the mastering stage and performance of the "I" seem to change. McDougall questions the "severe split between psyche and soma," and pays attention to the logic by which psychoanalysis supposes that bodily symptoms "were not revealed in the theaters of [...] mind. The curtains had been kept down, the words muffled" (McDougall, 1989, 2). Thus, interestingly, McDougall does not seem to conceive of psychoanalysis as a privileged tool for the "maintaining of meaning." She instead suggests what she calls "the psychosomatic potentiality," which is "part of every individual." This idea is already addressed in *Theatres of the Mind*, in which theater as a metaphor seems to be implicitly connected to an interest in *overcoming* the notion of the "normal," mastering "I":

> In taking the theater as a metaphor for psychic reality, I am hoping to avoid the standard psychiatric and psychoanalytic classification of clinical entities. Those terms apply to symptoms, not to people. To designate someone as a 'neurotic,' a 'psychotic,' a 'pervert,' or a 'psychosomatic' [...] implies that the rest of us are free of the psychic dramas that lie behind the symptoms to which these terms refer. [...] Each of us harbors in our inner universe a number of 'characters,' parts of ourselves that frequently operate in complete contradiction to one another, causing conflict and mental pain to our conscious selves. For we are relatively unacquainted with these hidden players and their roles. Whether we will it or not, our inner characters are constantly seeking a stage on which to play out their tragedies and comedies. Although we rarely assume responsibility for our secret theater productions, the producer is seated in our own minds [...]. (McDougall 1991, 3ff.)

Already in the theater of the mind, psychosomatic illness is presented as problematizing the idea of "mental stage production." The "psychosomatic theater" is said to be "the most dimly lit of the scenarios that belong to the psychic theater" because "the characters manage to put themselves on stage by profoundly altering the body's biological functioning" (McDougall, 1991, 11). In these scenarios, the soma is thought to "stage its own, essentially wordless, show" (McDougall, 1991, 11). "Psychosomatic dramas" differ from neurotic or psychotic mental dramas precisely because the latter "tell stories, and the key words of the plot may be deciphered eventually through the analytic process" (McDougall, 1991, 11). Thus, the telling of stories and the process of their deciphering seem to be contested by psychosomatic manifestations.

In *Theaters of the Body*, McDougall concludes that "[w]e all tend to somatize at those moments when inner or outer circumstances overwhelm our habitual psychological ways of coping" (McDougall, 1989, 3). McDougall relates these moments to the "pre-symbolic" phase of mother-child union, i.e., subject-object union, but we do not necessarily need to believe in these family narratives to acknowledge the interesting, uncanny relation between the bodily/material and the symbolic revealed here, the "hauntings" that McDougall associates with the acknowledgement of the *psychosoma*: "since its inception psychoanalysis, following Freud, has privileged the role of language in the structuring of the psyche and in psychoanalytic treatment. *But not all communications use language*" (McDougall,

1989, 11). Thus, McDougall argues that to contest the privileging of language ultimately means to challenge analysis itself, because "the psychosoma threatens to disrupt or evade the work of analysis" (McDougall, 1989, 11).

No Easy Access to the Psychosomatic Stage

Returning to the question of the visualizing function of theatrical metaphors, on the one hand, these metaphors of the theater allow audiences to "get a picture" or visualize the relations between the spheres of body and language, biology and psychology, pathology and the cultural/social/ethical/political, and finally, the sciences and the humanities. But on the other hand, the necessity for metaphorical language indicates the presence of something that cannot be described, explained, or comprehended *as such*, that there is a *problematic* moment, a lapse in both scientific explanation and hermeneutic understanding. While psychosomatics seems to highlight the fact that there is nothing "natural" about bodies and illnesses aside from cultural embeddedness, there seems to be paradoxically a certain counterforce of the bodily within and against the symbolic order and its privileging of language and rational meaning.

And thus we return to Schiller's *Robbers*. Stephanie Hammer's reading of Schiller's drama as a "theater of trauma," compares the play to the late twentieth-century graphic novel, which "provides the [...] equivalent of the German Storm and Stress drama": "Exaggerated, lurid, and rhetorically and visually over-the-top, [...] [comic] books propose a frame-by-frame performance of raw emotion—each cel [*sic*] representing a snapshot of a theater of the mind, to which the reader alone *has access*" (Hammer, 2001, 27; emphasis added). Hammer compares *The Robbers* to Neil Gaiman's *The Sandman*'s affective retelling of the traumatic Cain and Abel story. The point of connection would not primarily be the shared plot of the two rival brothers, but rather the means of visual and theatrical presentation. In the same way in which graphic novels impact their readers by "reintroducing the picture and the theatricality of *visible affect*" (Hammer, 2001, 28), Hammer argues, Schiller transforms the former attitude of distanced "pity" (for instance, in G.E. Lessing) "into a veritable explosion of violent empathy and identification" (20). This would explain why "Schiller's original audience fell into a hysterical frenzy at the end of the first production of his first play [*The Robbers*]" and why Peter Brooks "credits *The Robbers* as being the originator of European melodrama—a genre that works by undoing and crashing through all mechanisms of repression in order to create an experience of raw emotional affect. And the affect that Schiller himself stresses in the first production's playbill is *horror*" (Hammer, 2001, 20).

At first glance, this reading is tempting. If one believes—as psychoanalytic theory holds—that subjective experience is at its core traumatic, "the picture and the theatricality of *visible affect*" (Hammer, 2001, 28) would make this primal trauma *accessible*—less unfamiliar, more comprehensible, more communicable. However, we should keep in mind that any attempt to make affect visible—be it horror or despair, be it in graphic novels or in drama—detracts from "raw emotional affect" by the very attempt to make it *visible*. We must acknowledge that there is no such thing as horror or despair as a universal, un-situated category, but only this or that real or fictive person's horror and this particular—partial—attempt to make it somehow visible and accessible to oneself and/or others. Yet, Schiller explicitly points to this core ethical problem in visualizing affect in his medical dissertation, entitled *On the Connection Between the Animal and the Spiritual Nature in Man* (1780). There, he comments on his yet-to-be published first tragedy about the horror of affect:

> [Francis], heavily burdened with crimes, and once *crafty enough* in absolving all the sensations of humanity—by his skeleton-process—into nothing, now rises from a dreadful dream, pale and breathless, with a cold sweat upon his brow. [...] the spirit [struggling] with the horrors of the corporeal frame. ("Life of Moor," tragedy of Krake. Act. V. sc 1.). (Schiller, 2012, n. pag., emphasis added)

Gaining access to affect is a very dangerous game—Francis ends up being haunted or infected by the affects he himself "brought to stage" in the first place (in Act 2/Scene, mentioned above). It is he who ends up "pale as death" and "feverish," his "voice is [...] hesitating" (Schiller, 2014, Act V/Scene I).

Thus, going beyond and to some extent even *against* the long philosophical tradition in which "theater" served as a metaphor for "intelligible viewing" ("theater" descends etymologically from the Latin *thea*, "a view") in the context of psychosomatic discourse discussed here it rather highlights the limits of intelligibility, the limits or even dangers of an all too "crafty" attitude or desire. Subverting the notion of (over-)view, theater in these contexts emphasizes the partial, chaotic and de-centering pluri-mediality of verbal and non-verbal elements, of bodily and spatio-temporal aspects and insists on situatedness and disruption—on just *this* stage, just *this* gesture, body … Along the lines of Angela Woods's claim of "going beyond narrative," theatrical figures of thought would remind us that "the comforts of narrative—continuity, closure, and containment" only temporarily and apparently *triumph* over the again and again *problematic.* A critical and ethical reading of psychosomatics might borrow Francis's "hesitating voice" and resist winking at the still and enduringly unknown, unfamiliar, the paradoxical or ambiguous.

Bibliography

American Psychiatric Association. *Diagnostic and Statistical Manual of Mental Disorders: DSM-5*, 5th ed., American Psychiatric Association, 2013.

Aristotle. *Poetics*, translated by Malcom Heath, Penguin, 1996.

Didi-Huberman, Georges. *Invention of Hysteria Charcot and the Photographic Iconography of the Salpêtrière*, translated by Alisa Hartz, MIT Press 2003.

Dimsdale, Joel E., et al., "Somatic Symptom Disorder: An important change in DSM." *Journal of Psychosomatic Research*, vol. 75, 2013, pp. 223–228.

Dunbar, Helen Flanders. *Mind and Body: Psychosomatic Medicine*, Random House, 1966.

Ermann, Michael, et al., *Einführung in die Psychosomatik und Psychotherapie. Ein Arbeitsbuch für Unterricht und Eigenstudium*, 2nd ed., Kohlhammer, 2009.

Fitzgerald, Des, and Felicity Callard, "Entangling the Medical Humanities," in *The Edinburgh Companion to the Critical Medical Humanities,* edited by Anne White and Angela Woods, Edinburgh UP, 2016, pp. 35–49.

Foucault, Michel. "Polemics, Politics, and Problemizations," in *The Foucault Reader*, edited by P. Rabinow, Pantheon Books, 1984.

Foucault, Michel. "On Problematization," in *History of the Present*, vol. 4, 1988, pp. 16–17.

Frances, Allen. "New Disorder Risks Mislabelling Many as Mentally Ill." *BMJ: British Medical Journal*, vol. 346, no. 7900, 2013, p. 26.

Frank, Arthur W. *The Wounded Storyteller: Body, Illness, and Ethics*, U of Chicago P, 1995.

Freud, Sigmund. *The Standard Edition of the Complete Psychological Works of Sigmund Freud*, translated and edited by James Strachey, vol II (1893–1895): *Studies on Hysteria*, The Hogarth Press and the Institute of Psycho-Analysis, 1955.

Freud, Sigmund. "Abriß der Psychoanalyse," in *Gesammelte Werke*, vol. XVII: *Schriften aus dem Nachlass*, edited by Anna Freud, Imago Publishing, 1941, pp. 63–138.

Geisthövel, Alexa, and Bettina Hitzer, editors. *Auf der Suche nach einer anderen Medizin. Psychosomatik im 20. Jahrhundert*, Suhrkamp, 2019.

Greco, Monica. *Illness as a Work of Thought: A Foucauldian Perspective on Psychosomatics*, Routledge, 1998.

Hammer, Stephanie. *Schiller's Wound: The Theater of Trauma from Crisis to Commodity*, Wayne State UP, 2001.

Haraway, Donna. "A Cyborg Manifesto: Science, Technology, and Socialist-Feminism in the Late Twentieth Century," in *Simians, Cyborgs and Women: The Reinvention of Nature*, Routledge, 1991, pp. 149–181.

Harrington, Anne. *Mind Fixers: Psychiatry's Troubled Search for the Biology of Mental Illness*, W. W. Norton & Company, 2019.

Harrington, Anne. *The Cure Within: A History of Mind-Body Medicine*, W. W. Norton & Company, 2008.

Laplanche, Jean, and Jean-Bertrand Pontalis, *Das Vokabular der Psychoanalyse*, Suhrkamp, 2011.

Laplanche, Jean, and Jean-Bertrand Pontalis. *The Language of Psycho-Analysis*, W. W. Norton & Company, 1974.

Levenson, James L. *Textbook of Psychosomatic Medicine: Psychiatric Care of the Medically Ill*, 2nd ed., American Psychiatric Publishing Inc., 2011, pp. 295–298.

McDougall, Joyce. *Theaters of the Mind: Illusion and Truth on the Psychoanalytic Stage* [1982], Routledge, 1991.

McDougall, Joyce. *Theaters of the Body: A Psychoanalytic Approach to Psychosomatic Illness*, W. W. Norton & Company, 1989.

Macneill, Paul Ulhas. "The Arts and Medicine: A Challenging Relationship." *Medical Humanities*, vol. 37, 2011, pp. 85–90.

Mitscherlich, Alexander. "Zur Krise der Menschlichkeit in der Heilkunde [1948]." *Kranksein verstehen. Ein Lesebuch*, edited by Timo Hoyer, Suhrkamp, 2010, pp. 81–100.

Platner, Ernst. *Anthropologie für Aerzte und Weltweise*, Dyck, 1772.

Powell, Robert C. "Helen Flanders Dunbar (1902–1959) and a Holistic Approach to Psychosomatic Problems." *Psychiatric Quarterly*, vol. 49 no. 2, 1977, pp. 133–52.

Schiller, Friedrich. *The Robbers. A Tragedy*, 1781a, *Project Gutenberg*, Jul 20, 2014, https://www.gutenberg.org/files/6782/6782-h/6782-h.htm.

Schiller, Friedrich. *Die Räuber*, 1781b, *Sämtliche Werke*, vol. I, edited by Herbert Göpfert et al., DtV, 2004, pp. 481–618.

Schiller, Friedrich. "Philosophical Letters," 1780, *Project Gutenberg*, Nov. 6, 2012, https://www.gutenberg.org/files/6799/6799-h/6799-h.htm.

Schiller, Friedrich. "Versuch über den Zusammenhang der tierischen Natur des Menschen mit seiner geistigen," 1780, in *Sämtliche Werke*, vol. 5, edited by Herbert Göpfert et al., DtV, 2004, pp. 287–324.

Schings, Hans-Jürgen, editor. *Der ganze Mensch. Anthropologie und Literatur im 18. Jahrhundert*, Metzler, 1994.
Uexküll, Thure von. "Semiotics and Medicine." *Semiotica*, vol. 38, nos. 3–4, 1982, pp. 205–215.
Uexküll, Thure von. "Verwandlung seelischer Inhalte in körperliche Symptome," in *Grundfragen der psychosomatischen Medizin*, Rowohlt, 1963.
Viney, William et al. "Critical Medical Humanities: Embracing Entanglement, Taking Risk." *Medical Humanities*, vol. 41, 2015, pp. 2–7.
Weber, Samuel. "Psychoanalysis and Theatricality." *Parallax*, vol. 6, no. 3, 2000, pp. 29–48.
Weizsäcker, Viktor von. "Der Arzt und der Kranke: Stücke einer medizinischen Anthropologie," in *Gesammelte Schriften*, vol. 5, eds. Peter Achilles et al., Suhrkamp, 1987.
Whitehead, Anne, and Angela Woods, editors. *The Edinburgh Companion to the Critical Medical Humanities*, Edinburgh UP, 2016.
Woods, Angela. "Beyond the Wounded Storyteller: Rethinking Narrativity, Illness and Embodied Self-Experience," in *Health, Illness and Disease: Philosophical Essays*, edited by Havi Carel and Rachel Cooper, Acumen, 2012, pp. 113–128.
Woods, Angela. "The Limits of Narrative: Provocations for the Medical Humanities." *Medical Humanities*, vol. 37, 2011a, pp. 73–78.
Woods, Angela. "Post-narrative: An Appeal." *Narrative Inquiry*, vol. 21, no. 2, 2011b, pp. 399–406.

Reappropriating Breastfeeding as Power and Time in Photography and Feminist Discourse

Serena Fusco

Introduction: Global Promotion of Breastfeeding, Enduring Contradictions

> Ethnographic studies by social scientists have shown that breastfeeding throughout history and across different cultures is not only a nutritional exchange, but a complicated psychosocial cultural behavior. Tanya Cassidy and Abdullahi El Tom (2015)

This essay discusses and contextualizes three recent photoprojects on breastfeeding. Broadly speaking, all three can be placed in the context of a normalization and global-level promotion of breastfeeding that has been underway for at least three decades now. In July 1990, on the occasion of a

S. Fusco (✉)
Università degli Studi di Napoli "L'Orientale", Naples, Italy
e-mail: sfusco@unior.it

J. Cressman et al. (eds.), *Envisioning Embodiment in the Health Humanities*, Sustainable Development Goals Series,
https://doi.org/10.1007/978-3-031-49807-7_4

meeting in Florence, Italy, the Innocenti Declaration on the Protection, Promotion and Support of Breastfeeding was adopted by government policymakers from over thirty countries, setting an international agenda with ambitious targets for action. The Declaration was later endorsed by the forty-fifth World Health Assembly and the Executive Board of UNICEF (UNICEF Innocenti Research Center 2005). This is not to say that the road has since been smooth and that there is universal consensus on breastfeeding as a practice and on its meanings—far from it, in fact. Different opinions exist in different cultural contexts, as well as according to individual healthcare members, with regard, for instance, to its duration (how long it should last, and when it should be discontinued) or for how long it should remain the principal source of nutritional intake, with individual pediatricians often offering different recommendations. At the same time, the WHO and local governmental bodies promote breastfeeding as the ideal for newborns and very young humans. Breastfeeding is recognized as a public health matter, in the sense that its implementation has both short- and long-term benefits for human health—as a substantial body of medical scholarship argues. The WHO currently recommends breastfeeding on demand; six months of exclusive breastfeeding; the introduction of solid food ("complementary nutrition") at six months of age with human milk remaining the principal source of nutritional intake; and afterward, parallel to the assumption of appropriate solid foods, the continuation of breastfeeding until the child is at least two years old.[1] Both the U.S. and Italy—the two areas of the world where the photographers I discuss operate—have implemented their own national initiatives to increase breastfeeding rates in their population.

These recommendations and initiatives, however, exist amidst several unsolved contradictions and issues, including how to make WHO recommendations more than a desired but often—for practical reasons—unattainable goal. Acknowledging this recent and broadly consensual view of the importance of breastfeeding, *and simultaneously* paying attention to the nuances and often contradictory aspects that accompany this positive view, I will discuss three selected photoprojects and consider what strategies they use to represent breastfeeding. More specifically, I shall discuss whether (and how) these photoprojects depict breastfeeding as secluded, involving only a mother and a child, or, conversely; as involving other actors besides the mother and child; as happening in public spaces (or spaces endowed with public value); and/or as part of a "network" of relations rather than necessarily "dyadic." Eventually, the opposition between "dyad" and

[1] See WHO, "Breastfeeding: Recommendations."

"network" is shown to be much more of a *working* one, a heuristic distinction, than a substantial difference. The idea that breastfeeding always happens as part of an articulated network of social and cultural relations, and the conviction that breastfeeding has implications for social and cultural relations in a broad sense, constitute the culmination of my argument. The concept of "network" oscillates, in my usage, between, on the one hand, a recognition of the broad sociopolitical significance of breastfeeding, a practice that works as a "focal point" for many issues that revolve around it, and, on the other hand, a special appreciation of those forms of networking, of public and/or communitarian support that are based, first and foremost, on a recognition and a defense of the rights, power, agency, and desires of actually or potentially lactating women. The rights of a woman who possesses the power to lactate (as all women, with the exception of specific clinical conditions, do possess such power) also include, in fact, the right not to lactate. Last but not least, a claim for agency on the part of an always potentially lactating woman can involve, as we shall see, a claim for time beyond the well-ordered, clock-based, standardly shareable, regulated experience of it. While highlighting the differences among the photoprojects discussed, I shall consider all three in relation to the entwinement they create (albeit in different ways) between breastfeeding and time.

Photographic Renditions of Breastfeeding: Dyads, Networks, and How Time Matters

Francesca Cesari is a freelance photographer based in Bologna, Italy. According to her website, "[h]er artistic research focuses on people, mostly photographed in interiors with natural light. [...] The projects she leads concentrate on family, maternity, adolescence and human relationships."[2] The project *In the Room* comprises several photographs, each capturing what many would call, in a breastfeeding discursive context, a "dyad": a woman and a baby/child. Each photo is taken in a room, an interior space of which few details are revealed. The central theme of the project is breastfeeding, yet the specific focus is on breastfeeding as an act of accompaniment to sleep. Part of the photos capture the moment when the child is nursing; others capture a moment when the child is not at the breast anymore and is, instead, in the woman's arm, or propped on a shoulder, asleep after having nursed. The essential structure of each photograph is mother and child in an enclosed, recognizably private space.

[2] https://www.francescacesari.com/about/. Last accessed 21 August 2021.

The space forms a backdrop for the "dyad," which comes into visibility first and foremost in its mutuality and entanglement.

If, in Western culture, the visual rendition par excellence of the lactating woman is the *Madonna Lactans*,[3] Cesari's work can also be inserted into a visual context of reproduction, and possibly resignification, of this pictorial icon. *In the Room* explicitly builds, by means of an accumulation and juxtaposition of images, on the lactating Madonna icon, and on the archetype of the mother as life-giver (Oktober Matthews 2017). Despite their somatic differences, the portrayed women can be subsumed under a general "lactating woman" paradigm, also due to minimal presence of details which creates a very general sense of setting—a rocking chair, a couch, a window, a door frame, but not much else. A key element of all the images, more than the details of each room, is light itself—the way it falls upon and defines the bodies of woman and child in an almost Caravaggesque or Baroque fashion. Colors are also significant, further revealing Cesari's iconographic and stylistic research, which connect her photos to art history and how the pictorial arts have represented the act of nursing through the iconography of the *Madonna Lactans*. (Besides her training as a photographer, Cesari holds an MA in Art History.) In one of the pictures, an oversized door frame fleetingly evokes a museum space: this image may be read as a metavisual comment on the historical layers of artistic representation that set off the photographer's work. This intense reference to a pre-existing iconography is both meta-cultural *and* functional, I suggest, to establishing/reinforcing the "universal quality" of the lactating situation. The very reason for a public exposure of what happens "in the [private] room" seems to reside in this: "Despite this gentle act being everyday and universal, it still is often considered to be private, taking place only behind closed doors" (Oktober Matthews 2017).

I find it remarkable how Cesari's project openly engages time. The temporal—to an extent, I would suggest, *narrative*—structure of her project combines an iterative/cyclical pattern with a progressive/singulative one. If one of the key characteristics of the photographic medium is its capacity to capture a moment in time, Cesari makes this characteristic explicit by portraying a transitional moment by definition, one when mother and child are *suspended* between different states—namely, the child's transition from wakefulness into sleep and the nursing accompaniment thereof:

[3] See, among many possible references, the images discussed in Sperling (2016).

A secluded and silent place where a mother puts to sleep her child through breast-feeding.
The transition between waking and sleeping as the fulfillment takes over every resistance and distraction.
The mother's solid presence consciously supporting the baby's passage into unconsciousness,
renewing the ritual everlasting gestures of former generations.
A suspended moment of devotion and tenderness coexisting with the alienating repetitiveness of a routine. [...]

La dimensione appartata e silenziosa del luogo in cui una madre
addormenta il bambino attraverso l'allattamento al seno.
Il passaggio tra la veglia e il sonno dei piccoli, col progressivo ammorbidirsi del corpo
e l'abbandono di ogni resistenza, gioco e ostinazione.
La fisicità solida della donna, che accompagna con consapevolezza questa transizione
verso l'incoscienza e che rinnova i gesti rituali ed intuitivi delle generazioni che l'hanno preceduta.
Una parentesi sospesa dove la devozione e la tenerezza convivono con il risvolto alienante
di una routine che si ripete innumerevoli volte. (Cesari 2021)[4]

The transition from wakefulness to sleep is differently rendered in/through different images: some children (still) have their eyes open, others appear to have just closed them, others still have bodies that look "heavy" and abandoned in sleep. Understanding the moment of a child's transition into sleep is a delicate matter—as many caregivers, lactating or not, will know, laying down a baby who is not fully asleep will probably wake her/him up. For the viewers of the images, such transition keeps being "suspended" due to the different states of the children, some further along the transition, some less. A viewer moving through the exhibit will find no linear progression from wakefulness to sleep.

For the lactating woman, moreover, another layer of meaning is added. The endless repetitiveness of the ritual, the hint at "the ritual everlasting gestures of former generations," can be a token of its universal quality, but can also bring on a very human sense of alienation, and the issue is raised as to how this repetition can coexist with a (needed) renewal. Very

[4] https://www.francescacesari.com/in-the-room/. Last accessed 21 August 2021.

practically, a lactating mother can be divided between the tenderness and enjoyment of a single moment (or period) of nursing and the subtraction of enjoyment, and alienation, that comes from repetition. A temporal suspension is hence, from a lactating woman's perspective, also one between being ingrained in a repetitive mechanism that seems to allow no deviation, and the self-awareness that one can bring into this mechanism, possibly finding tenderness in it and, perhaps, a way to renew it. In temporal—even, as I have suggested, *narrative* terms—I find this series to be more complex than what can be perceived at first sight—also due to the potential for a photo series (as well as an exhibit) to be read and reread, creating renewed connections between the various discrete frames and, possibly, different "storylines" begotten by the accumulation or juxtapositions of readings and rereadings.[5]

More broadly speaking, such temporally and narratively charged suspension between repetition and renewal (a structure remindful of the opposition between the "pedagogical" and the "performative" that Homi Bhabha discussed a few decades ago) also speaks to breastfeeding as a highly intersubjective and broadly relational practice. Breastfeeding is "suspensive" also in the sense that, as soon as one starts to dig into its implications, one finds it inhering in many different discourses. Accordingly, breastfeeding has the potential to both reconfirm and disrupt such discourses. Among those—which I do not have the possibility to discuss in detail here—are old and new ideas of motherhood; the (female) body and its relation to science, medicine, and "nature"; the (female) body as (in)visible in private and public spaces; and the social and economic relevance of a human practice that is increasingly seen as a public health issue, but whose implementation is largely left to the resources and devices of individuals with goodwill, i.e., women who find themselves juggling different expectations and imperatives—as we shall presently see when discussing the other photoprojects. Discourses that revolve around lactation seem to coalesce in the private space of a room, yet they are inherently political; their bearing on the practice itself shows that lactation cannot be reduced, as it is too often the case, to a matter of purely individual choice or ir/relevance.

[5] On images as narrative, and on the possibility to read images according to different patterns depending on their patterns of exposure, see (among her rich work) at least Bal (1996) and (2009).

Moving across the Atlantic from Italy to the U.S., I am now going to discuss *Latched On*, a project by Gina Marie Brocker, a Boston-based documentary and wedding photographer. Presented on one of her two websites, *Latched On* has been published, in different versions, in several online sources.[6] Brocker's style is clearly different from Cesari's. In specifically visual terms, their expressive intent seems to be different, and their stylistic repertoire is also different. While the latter situates her project within an art-historical framework by referencing the iconography of the *Madonna Lactans*, the former's work can be situated in a discourse of documentary photography, one that tends to place its subjects in a detailed, recognizable environment and uses depth of field. The difference between Brocker and Cesari also evokes matters of genre: Brocker's work can more easily be ascribed to a genre that blends or alternates photographic elements with textual ones—namely, the photo-essay. I cannot enter into the debate around this photo-textual genre in the space of this essay; however, I wish to emphasize that the way in which words and photographs interact in Brocker's work exemplifies, in W.J.T. Mitchell's terms, a "dialectic of exchange and resistance between the [two mediums of] photography and language" (Mitchell 1994, 289) that is typical of the photo-essay at its best. As Mitchell argues, "The text of photo-essay typically discloses a certain reserve or modesty in its claim to 'speak for' or interpret the images; like the photograph, it admits its inability to appropriate everything that was there to be taken and tries to let the photographs speak for themselves or 'look back' at the viewer" (Mitchell 1994, 289). This entails an attempt at granting a space for the (often silenced) photographed subject(s) / subjects of discourse because of the partiality and limits that are inherent in both the photographic *and* textual component of the photo-essay.[7] This tentative network involves the mutual relations of at least three parties. Mitchell's discourse here reminds me of Ariella Azoulay's (later) idea of photography as an act in/of civil society, predicated on a potentially always open exchange between a photographer, (a) photographed subject(s), and the viewer of a photograph (see Azoulay 2008).

[6] See Brocker, *Latched On*; Brocker, "Breastfeeding"; and Brocker (2018).

[7] A crucial textual reference on the photo-essay—part of a seminal book on the word/image relationship—is Mitchell (1994), quoted above. On iconotexts and phototexts (including photo-essays) and their troubling function regarding what we consider "literature", see Cometa (2011) and (2016); on auto/biographical phototexts, see Coglitore (2014).

For my argument, what is especially relevant in Brocker's work—something that, besides the theme of breastfeeding *per se*, invites further comparison with Cesari's—is her handling of space and time. Brocker conveys various nuances of the public or semipublic in her photos, something that problematizes any given idea of breastfeeding as a fundamentally private act. This is also related to her choice of which people—besides the women and children—to include in the pictures. Several photographs do not exclusively portray the nursing "dyad"; to the contrary, they insert breastfeeding in a broader context, thus specifically creating a "breastfeeding situation," or a "network," situating lactation across what looks like a porous continuum between public and private spheres. "Talisa, Mackenzie & Max," for instance, features a "triad" seated at a table in a library, the mother simultaneously reading what we suppose is a folktale to the eldest child (a sign on a bookcase in the middle ground reads "folktales") and nursing the youngest. "Monica, Marlin & Simona," also featuring a "triad," is taken in a car parked on a public street: the woman nurses the youngest child and the eldest child sits close by. While the baby nurses in the crook of her arm, Monica holds reading material with one hand and sips from a plastic cup she holds in the other. "Kelly & Natalie," instead, is taken in a private space—the living room of a house or apartment, probably the featured family's home; it is a space wherein, though, the "public," external realm of work enters. A woman wearing a headset (headphones and mic) is typing on a laptop and breastfeeding a child who lies propped on her raised knee.

In my view, the way Brocker handles space has several implications. At one level, it thematizes the recurring issue of the visibility of breastfeeding, namely, the matter of how public—in this case, how *visible*—it can or should be; and it questions the idea that a private—i.e., domestic—space is the natural, or ideal, setting for breastfeeding. At another level, it also questions any easy dichotomy between public and private spaces, domestic and non-domestic, as we see a number of spaces where the two dimensions overlap: a car parked on the street; a living room doubling as an office space; an office as the space where another woman pumps her milk ("Robin"). Amanda Barnes Cook (2015) has suggested that "the 'public' of public breastfeeding […] generally refers to breastfeeding that occurs in the presence of other people, usually but not always outside of the home" (Barnes Cook 2015, 63):

> The "public" of public breastfeeding, in fact, often refers to spaces like the mall, the park, or restaurants—not places traditionally thought of as sites of public political importance. But, as feminists have maintained, women cannot be conceived of as equal peers in political and other important contexts if they are not treated as equals in the mall, the park, or restaurants—they cannot be equal participants in public deliberation and government if they cannot take up space in public without difficulty, if their concerns are chastised as being "inappropriate" for public forums. (Barnes Cook 2015, 64)

What Barnes Cook seems to suggest here is that the practice of lactation illuminates the public—here in the sense of *political*—value of a number of spaces that are not private but are not usually regarded as significant spaces for the definition and negotiation of the public sphere. Consistently with a long tradition of feminist thought and activism, the scope of what is political becomes expanded thanks to breastfeeding, if one considers what it means and what is implied, in terms of power relations, by the visibility of this practice when women exercise it as a public right and not as something to be concealed.

Brocker's declared intention is to create a *network*. "Hearing from the various caregivers reaffirmed how crucial sharing their experiences are. Knowing the realities of breastfeeding empowers families and normalizes this very natural and beneficial part of life" (Brocker, *Latched On*). Brocker herself, who had been nursing while working on her photoproject, is an invisible (because behind the camera) but peer component of it: "Usually worn in a wrap—and often nursing—my son, and later, daughter, and I ventured into over 50 Boston families' homes and lives to document their typical breastfeeding routines" (Brocker, *Latched On*). She is, in this project, a nursing mother among nursing mothers, despite being the one endowed with a camera. Her work is also remarkable in the way it documents (comparably to, but differently from, Cesari's series) the temporal dimension of breastfeeding and its perception on the part of both the photographed subject(s) and the photographer. In the words that accompany the images, at least two mothers comment on the power of breastfeeding to endow its participants with a gift of time beyond the usual limits:

> Nursing has, impossibly, gifted us more time […] I wish her little body would fit, soft and heavy, in my arms for always. Still, in the shade of her deepest sleeps, I can see her rosy mouth, eyes closed and head bobbing, as

> she anxiously searches for my breast. And time feels, for just a moment, a little more manageable. (Brocker, *Latched On*, "Danielle & Thea")

> What I love about it is the raw immediacy. A procrastinator and unplanner by nature, breastfeeding fits my lifestyle perfectly. Nothing to remember, nothing to clean just my ladies and my baby. Breastfeeding provides me with that sort of freedom and also empowerment. (Brocker, *Latched On*, "Monica, Marlin & Simona")

This exploration of time opens up interesting possibilities regarding the more general question of *how* one can conceive of time with relation to breastfeeding. Discourses of breastfeeding advocacy often raise the issue of time as the lactating mother's problem of reconciling the time for (outside) work and the time of domesticity. If the domestic space is regarded as the reign of full-time mothering and family care, it becomes especially hard to claim other forms of time; but the need is there, anyway. How about the breastfeeding mother (and, in an extensive logic, all mothers, *all* parents) wanting or needing to do something else entirely—like meeting a friend, or taking a walk? How about the right, the need, to have some time for oneself beyond the dichotomy between work and domesticity?

Can the practice of human lactation offer a possibility to reconsider time as a given? Can breastfeeding become a lens for focusing on temporalities that emerge, translucently, against the grain of a given temporal structure that has set itself, or has been set, as the organizing principle that orchestrates the flow of time? Take, for instance, "Kelly & Nathalie" (Brocker, *Latched On*) (Fig. 1). The situation portrayed in this photograph is highly ambivalent, in socioeconomic as well as temporal terms. For some breastfeeding advocates whose aim is to ensure the continuity of breastfeeding according to WHO standards at all costs, such a photo can represent victory: despite needing to work, the mother can, due to a "flexible" employment situation—working from home—continue to breastfeed her baby. She is not forced to interrupt breastfeeding because it is incompatible with her work schedule. On the other hand, this image can also be read in a less favorable light, i.e., as representing a condition—one that has been dramatically increased during the Covid-19 pandemic—in which the borders between

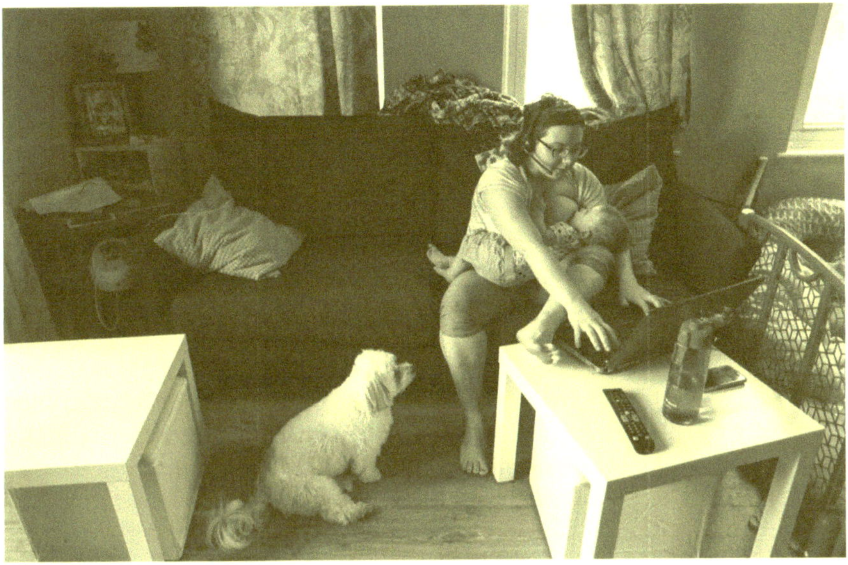

Fig. 1 Gina Brocker, "Kelly & Natalie", *Latched On*. (Courtesy of the artist. [Black and white from color original.] See the full project at http://www.ginamariebrocker.com/latched-on)

domestic space and workspace are increasingly being eroded, and a worker cannot count on a space or time that is really work-free. If it is possible to breastfeed while working—albeit in a rather uncomfortable physical position, like Kelly—why should women be granted work permits, or paid leave, in order to breastfeed (and work toward reaching the WHO breastfeeding goals)? Looking at such an image, one might ask whether the overlap of different times and spaces represented in Brocker's work can be read as an ipso facto endorsement of temporal and spatial fluidity, as a welcome questioning of clear-cut private/public dichotomies, as the opening of additional time windows, or, with less positive implications, as evidence not only of how capital maximizes work thanks to an increasing penetration into domestic spaces, but also of how women, lactating women included, are expected to be perfect and productive in all the aspects of their lives—as both paid workforce and hubs of domestic life.[8]

One of the paradoxes of breastfeeding nowadays is that, in a sociocultural context (and work condition) that regulates time by the clock and productivity by the ability to transform clock time into profit, we need to make time for lactation, i.e., to make time for a practice that seriously questions any attempt to attach it to both a schedule and productivity standards. And another enduring contradiction is that while breastfeeding on demand is the lactation practice that is nowadays recommended—as the one practice that can really work in the direction of prolonged and successful breastfeeding—many health professionals, and consequently many lay people, keep conceiving of breastfeeding in terms of "how many times a day" or "how many minutes per feeding," which often clashes with the reality of the experience. As Bernice Hausman notes, "[l]ucky is the mother whose doctor doesn't ask how often the baby feeds, since she might not be able to answer that question, or at least not satisfactorily to a physician who understands schedules to be the appropriate model of infant feeding" (Hausman 2003, 23).

To go back to our photographers: if in Cesari's work time is both cyclical and progressive, both pedagogical and performative, its structure both iterative and singulative, granting the possibility to make variations on a universalized theme, time in Brocker is more "reticular," due to the content and form of her photos, to their insertion into photo-essays, to the questions they raise and the connections they activate, whose ultimate aim is the practical construction of a support network for lactating women. I wish to emphasize, however, that practical, concrete objectives do not subtract from the theoretical potential that breastfeeding images can have.

[8]The issues that I raise here also speak to contemporary manifestations of what Rima Apple (2006) and Bernice L. Hausman (2003) call "perfect motherhood", i.e. the ideal, originating in the late nineteenth century, of a rational, science-based, and socially sanctioned way to raise one's children, at the best of one's abilities and at the same time looking at "objective" standards and striving to abide by them. During the past three decades or so, this struggle for perfection has taken on slightly different connotations (less "scientific" and more "nature-based") and has come to be known as "intensive motherhood". In Charlotte Faircloth's terms, "intensive motherhood" or "intensive mothering" is a form of "identity-work" that sees parenthood (with "parent" here being almost interchangeable with "mother") as an experience that is "financially, physically and emotionally intensive [...] parents are encouraged to spend a large amount of time, energy and money in raising their children. [...] [P]arenting is now an occupation in which adults (most typically, mothers) are expected to be emotionally absorbed and become personally fulfilled" (Faircloth 2009, 15).

In broad terms, it seems to me that both projects, albeit in different ways, attempt to elicit a gift of time from lactation.

Documenting various experiences of breastfeeding, Brocker attempts to create a sustaining narrative for nursing mothers, especially those who experience breastfeeding difficulties. The factual, contingent premise of several recent photo endeavors, especially those sponsored or co-sponsored by organizations that promote breastfeeding, is that, while the importance and benefits of breastfeeding are nowadays widely recognized, there is still, in many parts of the world, insufficient support for women who breastfeed. Several recent photoprojects, including Cesari's and Brocker's, follow a "breastfeeding normalization" agenda, i.e., they attempt to convey the message that breastfeeding can be performed by all women as an act of love that is natural to the human species.

Creating a support network around breastfeeding is an objective whose importance has recently been especially underlined and advocated by African American women in the U.S. A *Black Breastfeeding Week* has been organized since 2014, during which events are scheduled, meetings and debates held, and ideas exchanged on a peer-to-peer basis. Stressing the importance of creating a breastfeeding network for/around black women should not be understood as a separatist gesture, but instead as a way to address a recognized issue with roots in racial politics. According to journalist and initiative founder Kimberly Seals Allers, the reasons for adopting a race-based perspective on breastfeeding are grounded in fundamental disparities.

> *Black Breastfeeding Week* was created because for over 40 years there has been a gaping racial disparity in breastfeeding rates. The most recent CDC data show that 75% of white women have ever breastfed versus 58.9% of black women. The fact that racial disparity in initiation and even bigger one for duration has lingered for so long is reason enough to take 7 days to focus on the issue, but here are a few more: [...] (Seals Allers 2014)

Seals Allers lists additional reasons for implementing policies that may help boost breastfeeding rates among black women: a high black infant mortality rate; a high rate of diet-related diseases in black babies and children; a racial imbalance in breastfeeding advocacy, which is mostly white female-led; disregard for the culturally specific barriers that may prevent black women from breastfeeding; and lack of breastfeeding support in black-majority vulnerable communities (Seals Allers 2014).

Recent photographic work attempts to correct for the relative rarity of women of color's positive images of breastfeeding. The Chocolate Milk Mommies, a Birmingham-based group and nonprofit organization, has implemented several initiatives for decreasing racial disparity in access to health resources, an approach that includes raising awareness around breastfeeding and providing access to breastfeeding support for black women and communities.[9] Taking and circulating photographs of breastfeeding black women is one of the strategies employed by the group to raise awareness and draw support. According to an article published in *The Huffington Post* (Arboleda), the Chocolate Milk Mommies group was formed when several mothers answered an open call for a photo shoot to be realized during Black Breastfeeding Week. A second collective photo shoot, realized by photographer Lakisha Cohill, was highly successful, producing images that have been circulated through several publications and websites. The images include both portraits of individual mothers with their suckling babies and group portraits; all feature women and children in natural settings—woods, rocks, caves. The women, and sometimes the children, wear golden accessories like bracelets, necklaces, earrings, and especially hair ornaments that resemble crowns. Some of them pose holding a golden shaft topped by an Ankh symbol, thus evoking "the force of life" and harking back to an "African motherland." The women in these pictures have been described as impersonating "queens" or "goddesses": especially in the second case, a dimension of eternity, cyclical time, perhaps even timelessness, is evoked—a semantic field reinforced by the presence of the Ankh and the surrounding nature, with the caves gesturing toward prehistory, a time before time. This photoproject is grounded in the creation of a network, which, in turn, sets the stage for a series of photographic acts that (as it was the case for Brocker's work) connect the photographer and the photographed subjects: "Each woman represents a different chapter, including the one behind the lens" (Arboleda).

Photographic work like this black-centered project should be understood in the (historical) context of the peculiar perception of black women breastfeeding in the U.S. The issue of black breastfeeding sharply highlights what Bernice L. Hausman calls "the double bind of breastfeeding advocacy—an argument for breastfeeding as an empowering and healthful right of women and infants that typically devolves into an ideological view of proper mothering" (Hausman 2003, 71). Within a context of increased

[9] http://www.chocolatemilkmommies.org/about-us/. Last accessed 22 June 2021.

awareness regarding the health and social benefits of breastfeeding, women can be stigmatized for their infant feeding choices if one does not take into account the context wherein these choices are made. The lower rates of breastfeeding among black women can and sometimes result in faulting black women for not keeping up with the highest accepted health standards. On the other hand, in the highly influential study *At the Breast: Ideologies of Breastfeeding and Motherhood in the Contemporary United States* (1999), sociologist Linda Blum discusses the perspective of a group of working class black women who, she argues, turned away from breastfeeding as a self-conscious strategy for rejecting dominant representations of black female bodies, and to refuse the way their bodies had, for centuries, been associated with biological determinism, animality, exploitation on the part of others, and a lack of independence and self-determination. Blum here aptly de-naturalizes breastfeeding and reads it as part of a broader political discourse, emphasizing its use as a political tool—in this case, in the form of its strategic rejection.

While Blum neither explicitly advocates for breastfeeding nor starts from a consideration of its inherent importance, Hausman does both in her 2003 study *Mother's Milk: Breastfeeding Controversies in American Culture*. In further contrast with Blum, Hausman suggests that the lower rates of breastfeeding among black women may also indicate, instead of the result of a politically self-fashioning choice, "the medical establishment's inability to connect with black women's specific concerns about infant feeding and motherhood" (Hausman 2003, 219). Despite their different perspective on how to read the historically lower rates of black breastfeeding in the U.S., both Blum's and Hausman's studies are grounded in a belief that breastfeeding is a matter charged with cultural and political value in terms of both gender and race.

The Dyad in the Network: Concluding Remarks

As Blum argues, "[b]reastfeeding does not have inherent truth, but meanings determined out of power relations, various disciplining practices, and conflicting needs and interests, which are inherently political" (Blum 1999, 200). Both a biologically ingrained and a deeply cultural act, human breastfeeding has been endowed with changing meaning and ascribed with various significance in different historical and cultural contexts.[10] In the past as well as in the present, breastfeeding has been claimed by several discourses—medical, social, philosophical, cultural, artistic—and, probably because of such claims, despite being "natural," it yields conflicting interpretations and controversy. As Tanya Cassidy and Abdullahi El Tom write, "[t]he global community at the dawn of the twenty-first century [...] is looking to the life-saving properties associated with human lactation" (2015, 1–2). While there is now widespread consensus about the fact that breastfeeding must be facilitated for public health reasons—which include the demonstrated unique nutritional and immunological properties of mother's milk as well as the positive psychic aspects of the nursing relationship—this recognition is a recent phenomenon that is predicated on some historically complex factors. Accordingly, the currently renewed emphasis on the importance of breastfeeding needs to be historicized and put in perspective in its own terms.[11]

From a perspective that valorizes relationality as well as women's power *and* desire to breastfeed, pitting a "mother-centered" versus a "child-centered" conception of breastfeeding is highly questionable. Such an opposition is predicated on a problematic separation of "process" and "product" that cannot ultimately be held, because of the embodied nature of the breastfeeding relationship, and because milk, as shown by scientific research, is a substance that adjusts to the demands of the nursing party, who actively influences the quality and quantity of the milk produced: "insofar as breastfeeding is a condition or function of the maternal body that provides direct nutrition to offspring, there is no one subject—lactation describes a relation" (Hausman 2003, 192). For Van Esterik, since the breastfeeding relation is an ongoing and complex one, "[p]rocess language is better at capturing the embodied nature of nurturing experiences

[10] In the introduction to the collection *Medieval and Renaissance Lactations*, for instance, Jutta Gisela Sperling juxtaposes the meanings ascribed to human milk in ancient Greece versus ancient Rome, maintaining that "mother's milk was held in low esteem among ancient Greek physicians [...]. In contrast to the Greeks, who endowed breastfeeding with Dionysian promiscuity, magic powers, and maternal abjection, the Roman world never ceased to venerate goddesses in their capacity as both mothers *and* nurses" (Sperling 2016, 2, emphasis in the original).

[11] Synthetic and convincing historical reconstruction can be found in Hausman (2003, 6–15) and Wolf (2006, 404–409). An especially interesting historical factor is the entwinement between "science" and "nature" that has characterized the promotion of breastfeeding since the late nineteenth century.

like breastfeeding; the complex symbiotic relation between mother and infant has communication and co-regulation functions that extend far beyond nutrition. [...] [I]t is near impossible to separate the effects of the product, human milk, from the process of breastfeeding" (Van Esterik 2015). I would also observe that emphasizing the lactating woman's desire, control, and intrinsic power and right to lactate means to value her active relationship with the nursing party—be it her biological child or not, like in the case of other lactation possibilities.[12] However, such a relationship must not necessarily be symbiotic in the sense of being exclusive. While lactation often occurs in a room, it must not be constrained there. Starting from the awareness of a nursing *relationality* sheds light on how a woman can exercise her power in order to transform the (sociopolitical) conditions that deprive her of the power to lactate, and establish such a relation, when she wishes to. In other words, the dyad (Cesari) makes sense precisely to the extent that it is always already (actually or potentially) inserted in a network (Brocker, Cohill). In practical terms, the creation of a peer network for sustaining breastfeeding supports the idea of breastfeeding as (inherently) intersubjective, not only in the sense of being a communication channel for the mother/child dyad, but also a space of exchange and an opportunity for a broader community (Frampton 2004; Wolf 2006).

The idea that milk creates kinship is an ancient one. Terms like "milk sisterhood" or "milk brotherhood" are well known; in some legal systems of the past, an incest taboo was established between illicit lovers by having the man drink the woman's milk. Aunchalee Palmquist (2015) highlights the "kin-like affinities" (40), the molding and shaping of social bonds through the web-powered recent phenomenon of informal milk sharing. One of the quotes in her essay, from one of the Facebook pages that bring together different subject who share (give and/or receive) human milk, highlights milk sharing as a networking practice that goes in the direction

[12] Fiona Giles discusses other scenarios, such as adult nursing, lactation eroticism, and male attempts at lactation. Giles attempts to disconnect breastfeeding from its privileged connection with both womanhood and motherhood, seeing it (in material, not merely symbolic terms) as a way to question gender and sexual binarisms and promote "fluid subjectivities" and reciprocity in relations (Giles 2005). Giles also underlines the emotional, non-strictly nutritional function of nursing, and here she is in good company, as the medical profession itself has come to underline the breastfeeding relation as one of care and bonding well beyond nutrition—a bond that is, though, usually made to coincide with the mother-child bond, a perspective that Giles attempts to expand.

of creating a kind of intersubjectivity that empowers all lactating subjects, including the women who have unjustly come to doubt the power of their own bodies: "We can foresee a time when women protect each other and help one another feed their babies so that every mother feels whole and no mother feels broken or that her body is failing her" (qtd. in Palmquist 2015, 34). One of the most interesting features of Palmquist's study is that it situates the practice of informal milk sharing "at the intersection of medicalization and demedicalization" (Palmquist 2015, 39):

> Medicalized breastfeeding discourses are almost always constructed around the definition that breastfeeding is a biological act of motherhood, which is confined to her biological offspring. Milk sharing challenges the idea that breastfeeding and feeding breastmilk is the sole domain of women and mothers. Fathers and other caregivers whose roles, sex, and gender identities do not conform to hetero-normative standards now have greater access to breastmilk. Milk sharing enables them to enact emergent identities and create novel expressions of caregiving that unsettle the notion that breastfeeding and feeding breastmilk is strictly a womanly art. (Palmquist 2015, 43)

Subjective and objective dimensions here intertwine, and science becomes infused with the need to empower individual women, helping them regain control of their female bodies via the nursing function. The scope of the discourse broadens here *beyond the womanly body per se*, giving another twist to the long-standing feminist idea of embodiment. Literally in cases of milk-sharing, practically *and* rhetorically in the projects I have discussed in this essay, the embodied nursing function extends, network-like, beyond the mother-child dyad.

Bibliography

Apple, Rima D. *Perfect Motherhood: Science and Childrearing in America*. Rutgers UP, 2006.

Arboleda, Cindy. "This Empowering Photo Shoot Aims to Normalize Breastfeeding In The Black Community." *The Huffington Post. U.S. Edition*. https://www.huffpost.com/entry/thisempowering-photo-shoot-aims-to-normalize-breastfeeding-in-the-black community_n_5a21b1bee4b03c44072d7fd9. Last Accessed 21 August 2021.

Azoulay, Ariella. *The Civil Contract of Photography*. Zone Books, 2008.

Bal, Mieke. *Narratology: Introduction to the Theory of Narrative*. 3rd edition. U of Toronto P, 2009.

———. *Double Exposures: The Subject of Cultural Analysis*. Routledge, 1996.

Barnes Cook, Amanda. *Breastfeeding, Feminism, and Political Theory*. PhD diss., University of North Carolina at Chapel Hill, 2015.

Blum, Linda. *At the Breast: Ideologies of Breastfeeding and Motherhood in the Contemporary United States*. Beacon Press, 1999.

Brocker, Gina Marie. *Latched On: The Realities of Breastfeeding*. http://www.ginamariebrocker.com/latched-on/. Last Accessed 21 August 2021.

———. "Breastfeeding." *Lens Culture*. https://www.lensculture.com/projects/371820-breastfeeding. Last Accessed 21 August 2021.

———. "The Realities of Breastfeeding Today—A Photo Essay." *Motherly*, August 23, 2018. https://www.mother.ly/life/the-realities-of-breastfeeding-today-a-photo-essay. Last Accessed August 21, 2021.

Cassidy, Tanya, and Abdullahi El Tom. "Introduction." *Ethnographies of Breastfeeding: Cultural Contexts and Confrontations*. Edited by Tanya Cassidy and Abdullahi El Tom. Bloomsbury, 2015. Kindle ed., pp. 1–10.

Cesari, Francesca. 2021. *In the Room*. https://www.francescacesari.com/in-the-room/. Last Accessed 21 August 2021.

Coglitore, Roberta. "I dispositivi fototestuali autobiografici. Retoriche e verità." *Between*, vol. 4, no. 7, 2014, pp. 1–37.

Cometa, Michele. "Forme e retoriche del fototesto letterario." *Fototesti. Letteratura e cultura visuale*. Edited by Michele Cometa and Roberta Coglitore. Quodlibet, 2016, pp. 69–115.

———. "Fototesti. Per una tipologia dell'iconotesto in letteratura." *La fotografia. Oggetto teorico e pratica sociale*. Edited by Vincenza Del Marco and Isabella Pezzini. Nuova Cultura, 2011, pp. 63–101.

Faircloth, Charlotte. "Mothering as Identity-Work: Long-Term Breastfeeding and Intensive Motherhood." *Anthropology News*, February, 2009, pp. 15–17.

Frampton, Edith. "Fluid Objects: Kleinian Psychoanalytic Theory and Breastfeeding Narratives." *Australian Feminist Studies*, vol. 19, no. 45, 2004, pp. 357–368.

Giles, Fiona. "The Well-Tempered Breast: Fostering Fluidity in Breastly Meaning and Function." *Women's Studies*, vol. 34, 2005, pp. 301–326.

Hausman, Bernice L. *Mother's Milk: Breastfeeding Controversies in American Culture*. Routledge, 2003. Kindle ed.

Mitchell, W.J.T. "The Photographic Essay: Four Case Studies." *Picture Theory: Essays on Verbal and Visual Representation*. The U of Chicago P, 1994, pp. 281–322.

Oktober Matthews, Katherine / GUP Team. "In the Room." *GUP* 7 July 2017. https://gupmagazine.com/portfolios/in-the-room/. Last Accessed 21 August 2021.

Palmquist, Aunchalee. "Demedicalizing Breastfeeding: The Discourses, Practices, and Identities of Informal Milk Sharing." *Ethnographies of Breastfeeding:*

Cultural Contexts and Confrontations. Edited by Tanya Cassidy and Abdullahi El Tom. Bloomsbury, 2015. Kindle ed., pp. 23–44.

Seals Allers, Kimberly. "Top Five Reasons We Need A Black Breastfeeding Week." *Black Breastfeeding Week* 19 August 2014. https://blackbreastfeedingweek.org/why-we-need-black-breastfeeding-week/. Last Accessed 21 August 2021.

Sperling, Jutta Gisela. *Medieval and Renaissance Lactations: Images, Rhetorics, Practices*. Routledge, 2016. Kindle ed.

UNICEF Innocenti Research Center. "1990–2005. Celebrating the Innocenti Declaration on the Protection, Promotion, and Support of Breastfeeding: Past Achievements, Present Challenges and the Way Forward for Infant and Young Child Feeding." UNICEF, 2005. https://www.unicef-irc.org/publications/pdf/1990-2005-gb.pdf. Last Accessed 21 August 2021.

Van Esterik, Penny. "Foreword. What Flows Through Us: Rethinking Breastfeeding as Product and Process." *Ethnographies of Breastfeeding: Cultural Contexts and Confrontations*. Edited by Tanya Cassidy and Abdullahi El Tom. Bloomsbury, 2015. Kindle ed. No page reference.

WHO, "Breastfeeding: Overview." https://www.who.int/health-topics/breastfeeding#tab=tab_1. Last Accessed 14 August 2021.

———. "Breastfeeding: Recommendations." https://www.who.int/health-topics/breastfeeding#tab=tab_2. Last Accessed 14 August 2021.

Wolf, Jacqueline H. "What Feminists Can Do for Breastfeeding and What Breastfeeding Can Do for Feminists." *Signs: Journal of Women in Culture and Society*, vol. 31, no. 2, 2006, pp. 397–424.

Enactment, Entanglement, #Endometriosis: Feminist Technoscience and the Instagrammatic Illness Narrative

Amanda K. Greene

Introduction

Endometriosis is an illness of knots and tangles, of bindings and border-crossings. Endometrial tissues grow, develop, and spread outside of their "appropriate" womb-bound confinement, connecting apparently disparate parts of the body; uterine cells migrate as far as the lungs or wrap around nerves to cause radiating pain down the legs; adhesions bind organs together into new assemblages (Hummelshoj 2018). The Instagrammatic illness narrative is a similarly tangled phenomenon. Social media affordances and quotidian user posting practices bring different manifestations of illness—from fecal samples to selfies—together into new hybrid configurations. In spite of the neat lines of separation suggested by

A. K. Greene (✉)
Center for Bioethics and Social Sciences in Medicine, University of Michigan Medical School, Ann Arbor, MI, USA
e-mail: akgreene@umich.edu

J. Cressman et al. (eds.), *Envisioning Embodiment in the Health Humanities*, Sustainable Development Goals Series,
https://doi.org/10.1007/978-3-031-49807-7_5

Instagram's signature squarely gridded format, illness narratives on the platform are composed of ever-evolving, tightly knitted connections that resist stabilization into discrete events or singular, unified phenomena. Social media is a way of "doing" illness on an everyday basis as material bodies extend into virtual space and digital cultures simultaneously migrate into physical objects, flesh, and cells outside of the platform's bounds.

This chapter argues that a critical feminist framework is well-situated to grapple with how "wounded storytelling" (Frank 2013) unfolds on visual social media without artificially unraveling the complex hybridities that define these narratives. By leveraging two major theories from this scholarly tradition—enactment and entanglement—to examine a number of accounts and posts clustered around #endometriosis on Instagram, my intervention suggests how feminist technoscience can generatively shape health humanities research on today's dynamic digital cultures. Feminist technoscience and research on illness narratives have had surprisingly little overlap, with the notable exception of a 2018 special issue of *Catalyst: Feminism, Theory, Technoscience* on "Illness Narratives, Networked Subjects, and Intimate Publics."[1] Yet, as digital contexts increasingly demand alternative theoretical frames that live at the interface of human bodies and new technologies, this scholarly nexus can be an invaluable resource for the twenty-first-century health humanities. Approaches that integrate feminist technoscience into the already rich body of work on illness narratives offer more nuanced perspectives than approaches that focus on how digital culture updates earlier forms of discourse. Furthermore, this critical orientation can sidestep the impulse to understand online narratives as primarily virtual constructions that simply *represent* illness by instead tracing new media deep into the flesh.

* * *

Endometriosis occurs when endometrial tissue grows outside of the uterus. The medical community indicates that this condition impacts approximately one in ten women during their reproductive years, but non-binary individuals are also affected. A wide assortment of symptoms is possible, depending on which organs are affected, but the most

[1] The six articles testify to the richness of combining feminist technoscience, digital culture, and illness narratives. I hope to build on this corpus of work in a way that foregrounds potentially transferable methods and that emphasizes the visual multimodalities of Instagram.

consistent sign of endometriosis is severe pain. Unfortunately, in spite of the prevalence of this condition and the severity of its symptoms, many medical professionals see these signs as a psychological issue or an overreaction to "bad period pain" (Denny 2004; Jones 2016). As a result, 46% of endometriosis patients see more than five doctors before being diagnosed and diagnosis takes an average of eight years from the initial onset of symptoms (Ballweg 2004). While there is still no cure for endometriosis, timely diagnosis can facilitate pain management strategies and access to medications that limit endometrial tissue growth, or surgical excisions to remove particularly invasive manifestations.

There are a number of reasons why the endometriosis community makes an ideal case study for this feminist approach to online illness narratives. On the one hand, the illness's own entangled form and individuals' engagement with its messy physiological manifestations intensify features of the Instagrammatic illness narrative that exist across other conditions as well. Less abstractly, too, endometriosis has been at the heart of recent debates about contested knowledge-making in medical contexts and, especially, the dismissal of female experiences of pain.[2] It evokes a long history of female-focused (mis)treatment revolving around hysteria—both via the notorious concept of the wandering womb and later when endometriosis's physical symptoms were considered part of a hysterical conversion disorder.[3] Furthermore, endometriosis problematizes the medical gaze in ways that make individual narrative practices especially urgent. Currently, a clinical diagnosis can only be officially confirmed by laparoscopic surgery. Many women who are treated for endometriosis or suffer symptoms never have this procedure due to cost or because medical providers deem it unnecessary. But even for those who do have the surgery, this technological diagnostic is limited because there is little correlation between how endometriosis is enacted by the visual signs in this procedure and the intensity of symptoms experienced by the patient (Porpora et al. 1999). Institutional lacunas prompt intensive self-narrativization and self-diagnosis to fill gaps in recognition, naming, and meaning-making, which fosters a vital and active culture of online storying around endometriosis experiences (Culley et al. 2013; Markovic et al. 2008; Whelan 2003).

[2] For a recent popular example see Norman, *Ask Me About My Uterus* (2018).

[3] See Wilson *Psychosomatic* (2004) for more on hysteria and conversion disorder.

Narrative and Illness

Health humanities scholarship has influentially challenged the notion that disease can be defined solely by its diagnostic criteria. Kleinman's (1988) work in the 1980s was a fundamental step in articulating that illness is not simply an accumulation of symptoms or tissue damage but is defined by patients' experiences and sociocultural contexts. Frank's later (2013) theorization of the "wounded storyteller" extended this work to stress how different modes of storying can deeply change patients' experiences. Frank emphasizes that "ill people learn by hearing themselves tell their stories, absorbing others' reactions and experiencing their stories being shared," and that this learning materially impacts their understandings and the trajectories of their illness. Newer investigations of illness narratives *online* have built on this foundation and demonstrated considerable continuity with earlier scholarship on the value of narrative in aiding patients' understanding and agency in relation to their illness. For example, Ressler et al.'s study (2012) of patients who blogged about their illness experience found that blogging created opportunities for them to make meaning and gain insights into their illness in addition to creating accountability to oneself and others.

While the bulk of this work examines the forums and blogs that defined digital communications in a pre-social media era, the blogosphere is no longer representative of today's extensive ecosystem of digital communication. Social media has become the key site where illness stories are generated online, and activity on these networked, multimodal platforms often reshapes conventional narrative models more than blogs. In addition to the new affordances that social media platforms provide, social media reaches wider user-bases and is used more frequently than earlier iterations of online storytelling. According to the Pew Research Center, in 2021, 72% of U.S. adults used at least one social media site. This share is even higher among younger demographics. For example, one recent study indicated that "more than nine in ten (93%) teens and young adults report using social media [...] 81% say they use it on a daily basis, including 17% who say they use it 'almost constantly' and 54% who do so multiple times a day" (Rideout and Fox 2018). As social media usage has become a ubiquitous part of everyday experience, the stories told on these platforms have adapted to these new circumstances.

The limited number of studies of illness narratives on social media have consistently identified ways in which digital storying is formally distinct from the narratives produced via older media forms. For example, Han and Wiley (2013) emphasize how the more interactive nature of social media leads to a "new form of health communication," by shifting patients toward conversation instead of one-way narrative. Likewise, Arduser (2017), in a study of diagnosis vlogs on YouTube, directly claims that social media "remediates" the idea of diagnosis along with how it is related.[4] Gonzalez-Polledo and Tarr's (2016) comprehensive examination of how individuals communicate pain on Tumblr and Flickr highlights how the visual affordances of platforms impact narrative form. Illness narratives drift away from conventional arcs on social media platforms and instead hinge on momentary affective evocations that need not add up to a cohesive story. For example, a "pain meme" relies on popular culture to reframe the idea of pain in ways that are legible to an online community; such modes of storying create online "pain worlds" and serve as shibboleths that enable insiders to enter these spaces as opposed to mimetically reflecting individuals' experiences over time.

As these scholars stress, social media undeniably changes what illness narratives look like. But such changes are not confined to user posts and online interactions. Equally important are the myriad ways in which these narratives spill outside of the affordances of particular platforms, constituting expansive narrative ecologies that blend online and offline worlds. Social media storytelling does not only alter narrative form but also alter how the body is wrapped up in these forms. While Gonzalez-Polledo (2016) gestures briefly at the fact that "online devices are also changing what it means to live with chronic illness," this line of analysis demands more attention. The transformation of the illness narrative is not just about how illness is represented but how it is felt and lived. Starting from feminist technoscience offers a way of engaging with the novelties of the Instagrammatic illness narrative head-on, in ways that are not entrenched in what Jurgenson (2012) has termed "digital dualism" and that are go beyond comparative engagements rooted in how new media "updates" older models of storytelling.

[4] Remediation, forwarded by Bolter and Grusin (2000), refers to the ways in which new media adapt and reproduce the form and content of older media.

Feminist Technoscience

Feminist technoscience is a rich and eclectic field that uses critical feminist thought to consider the sociocultural dimensions of technologies and scientific frameworks. This work frequently problematizes stable categories and fixed identities—illuminating the blurring of culture and biology, as well as the importance of contextualized, situated modes of knowledge production. Haraway's (2003) hybrid notion of "natureculture" is emblematic of this theoretical approach. Like much of Haraway's work, natureculture captures the impossibility of maintaining clean distinctions between apparently binary concepts. Pushing against common discussion of nature versus nurture, or biology versus social construction, natureculture encapsulates the complex ways in which these categories are fundamentally bound up with one another and impossible to disentangle. To use a more concrete example, Fausto-Sterling (2005) has examined the ways in which even phenomena that may appear purely physiological at first glance, like bones, are both biological and cultural. As she argues, although bones in women are not inherently more prone to osteoporosis, cultural norms that limit girls' rough physical activity have material impacts on the physical composition and health of their bones. Such cases show how, in her words, bodies "physically imbibe culture" (p. 1495).

I will focus on two separate, important theoretical terms that have emerged from the tradition of feminist technoscience and that mesh particularly well with conversations in the health humanities—enactment and entanglement. While neither concept is explicitly concerned with narrative (and as a result has not been a prominent part of work in this area) they can help trace the ways online accounts exist as material modes of accounting for illness that act on and through users' bodies. I will gloss these terms, illustrate how they fit into discussions about social media illness narratives, and trace them through accounts by four different users in the Instagram endometriosis community who have given me permission to discuss and reproduce their posts.[5] This analysis sheds light on feminist technoscience's underexplored symbiosis with narrative-focused health

[5] I identified these accounts by examining a large dataset of posts tagged with #endometriosis, collected with the University of Amsterdam's Digital Methods Initiative's open-source hashtag explorer. From this preliminary corpus, several particularly rich, representative, and active accounts were identified to serve as exemplary cases. The owners of these accounts were contacted via email or Instagram Direct Message in order to request permission to analyze and reproduce their posts in this scholarship.

humanities scholarship, and the ways the nexus of these two scholarly traditions can inform future research by helping scholars embrace emergent complexities of envisioning ill embodiment on and offline.

Enactment: The Body Multimodal

In her influential *The Body Multiple* (2002) Mol argues that illness is not a concrete thing that exists within the body but instead a dynamic activity: "illness is something being done to you, the patient. And something that, as a patient, you do" (20). Mol emphasizes that this "doing"—which she terms enactment—brings illness ontologically into being. Illness not only is "done," but, even more importantly, only exists through this doing; illness is not "merely" practiced as opposed to "really existing" in a material way. Enactments include patients' conscious performances and doctors' official diagnoses but are also produced by a multitude of other human and non-human agents. Illness is done by organs, medical knowledge, diagnostic technologies, and more. The case study Mol uses to elaborate on her theory focuses on the enactment of atherosclerosis in the Netherlands. In this research, she demonstrates how multiple *atheroscleroses* are constituted by medical imaging, by autopsy data, by a patient's habits of walking, by descriptions of symptomatic pains, etc. Illness is not something hidden inside the body that can be fully revealed by medical instruments or that is represented by patients' descriptions of their ailments. Technology, narrative, and physiology are all different ways in which illness is brought into being and "done."

Posts within the Instagram endometriosis community mirror the range of the enactments that Mol highlights in her monograph. It is especially notable how frequently users call on imaging technologies that help construct their endometriosis in their accounts. For example, many share ultrasounds and laparoscopic images that were generated to define and deal with the illness in clinical spaces. Other posts enact the illness with photographs of the litany of medications that users take on a daily basis to manage or treat their symptoms. Captions that accompany these images frequently reinforce the medication's status as agents that are "doing" endometriosis. For example, a photograph of prescription pill bottles by @ the1in10woman is accompanied by the text "my 'invisible illness,'" suggesting that the medications are visible evidence of her endometriosis and are thus key players in enacting the illness as opposed to contextual details. By highlighting the invisibility of the illness on the surface of their bodies, users draw attention to the many ways in which illness is practiced or done, instead of something that can be found on (or even in) the body. To offer another example, @endospoon posts ultrasound images accompanied by a narrative about diagnosis in the caption. As she recounts, these medical images of her uterus are synonymous with endometriosis coming into being in her life, coalescing embodied experiences of pain into a named, clinically recognizable entity. But the images are not simply provided as proof of the reality of her illness. Instead, as her story emphasizes, they are part of a larger ecosystem in which her endometriosis is done as opposed to capturing what "really is" and superseding the value of her symptomatic pain and other parallel enactments.

When illness is enacted by so many different actors, multiple versions of illness and the body exist simultaneously and in tension. In Mol's words, if we "shift to studying bodies and diseases while they are being enacted in daily hospital practices, multiplication follows." On Instagram, the body multiple is particularly visible and important to the doing of illness because of the platform's *multimodality,* which strikingly magnifies the immediate impression of multiplicity. Multimodality refers to the blending of multiple forms of communication (text, sound, images, video, etc.) that has come to characterize much of our digital media environment. Critically, multimodal narrative forms are more than the sum of their parts; multimodal communication demands literacies that span all the modes employed as well as an understanding of how these multiple modes interact when assembled together.

It is worth stressing that in the Instagram endometriosis community, this multimodal multiplicity also occurs within individual accounts. Users frequently juxtapose clinical diagnosis, medication, informational pamphlets, autobiography, news stories, popular media, their own bodies, artwork, etc. While Mol writes that "the stories people tell [about their illness] do not just produce grids of meaning," Instagram's signature grid of square images makes it unusually visibly clear how an individual's endometriosis is enacted by a wide range of actors and is constituted simultaneously by various different technologies of seeing and forms of knowing (15). Indeed, this multiplicity is not an abstract theoretical construct but part of how users themselves deliberately make meaning and communicate the many endometrioses they live and encounter on a daily basis.

A glance at @emlwy's account, for example, displays a multitude of endometrioses coexisting within even a brief slice of a single account.[6] Her posts combine many of the same sorts of enactments described above, drawing on food, medication, hashtags, blogs, inspirational quotes, selfies, and more. Although the self-portrait with the #1in10 sign or the photograph of medication are very different modes of enacting illness than the simple text "please don't make a pregnancy joke" these entries are all doing endometriosis. Such multiplicity defines Instagrammatic illness narratives at all scales, even in single posts. Zooming in on one of @emlwy's posts demonstrates the same reliance on various distinct yet intertwined enactments that characterizes her account as a whole: the photographed fecal sample, processes of scientifically analyzing the sample, her fecal matter itself, the diagnostic results from the colonoscopy, her conversation with the doctor, her written description of her experience. Even at the level of the single word, her collage of hashtags is another mode in which endometriosis is enacted and multiplied online; #endometriosis is a means of enacting illness by claiming and naming it. The way tags like #hysterectomy, #endosisters, #ischemiccolitus, and #healthblogger are linked together offers a window into her endometriosis as it is dynamically done in dialogue with multiple actors inside and outside of the body—from her colon to health blogging culture—as opposed to being a single diagnosable thing.

Another important piece of Mol's argument is her insistence that the body multiple does not fall apart in spite of its radical multiplicity. Forms of coordination and distribution ease over contradictions and help maintain body and illness as cohesive wholes. In the hospital, norms, regulations, and hierarchies of knowledge-production enable coordination, but in virtual space (not to mention in the case of contested diagnoses and invisible illnesses) that body is more tenuous. While users do frequently bring in healthcare providers and clinical environments as actors, other enactments don't automatically cede their authority as in Mol's account. In the case of endometriosis and on social media, in the absence of clear institutional authority, the online illness narrative serves as a key scaffolding that manages the multiplicity of the body just as it helps the diverse modes of storying hold together in a single account.

On Instagram, individuals coordinate the multiplicity of their illness experiences through an embrace of multimodal storytelling that integrates

[6] https://www.instagram.com/explore/tags/emlwy/

different literacies and modes of meaning-making. Envisioning the body multimodal on social media facilitates the coordination of a chronically ill body that threatens to fall apart in the face of cyclical experiences of crip time that evade curative narratives and conventional containment by the medical system. Although multimodality frequently appears natural or familiar in a digital world, that does not mean its usage should be taken for granted. Individuals have control over how multimodal their own social media posting practices are, and these communication choices have important consequences on how content is narrated and experienced. Social media is thus not just a narrative venue but a site where the body is made and managed; it offers a consistent mode of coping with the potentially fragmenting pressures of illness enactments that can't be meshed.

The coordination just described is also facilitated by narrative practices that anchor multiplicity to legible genres and tropes that can meaningfully sustain an unwieldy range of expressions, curating a holistic experience available to larger communities. Melander's (2019) examination of the striking multimodality of one exemplary endometriosis Instagram account highlights the nested structures that hold individual posts together and, in so doing, help maintain the coherence of the body multiple. As she synthesizes, "by means of visual and verbal resources, separate posts thus appear to be embedded in three ways; in relation to the ongoing personal story, in relation to the account, and in relation to the typical or larger narrative about endometriosis" (Melander 87). This latter relationship is both particularly important online and facilitated by social media platform architectures. Connection to a larger narrative about endometriosis that exceeds the individual is facilitated by common anchors from a range of cultural contexts that exceed the platform—definitions from organizations that raise awareness about the illness, books or documentaries about endometriosis, or even meaningful blog posts. Touchstones translate the enactment of endometriosis beyond personal experience and into forms that are familiar within the context of this online community. They also help quilt together the potentially disparate content that constitutes these social media accounts. Shared sources and rhetorical tropes within individual posts and speckled across accounts are one key to coordinating endometriosis in the absence of a clinical authority and clearly demarcated clinical spaces. Even a single hashtag can serve this purpose, as it fixes individual experience in relation to something "real" and other validating communities.

Returning to @emlwy's account, the posts regularly anchor her individual embodied life to circulated structures of meaning-making attached to a variety of communities and authorities. Cultural tropes and texts such as a Maya Angelou quote or the #1in10 poster are signposts that help ground more personal or decontextualized enactments of endometriosis that might not be so immediately legible or communicable to outside readers. Indeed, the #1in10 post is a particularly clear, common example. The hashtag itself began as part of an awareness campaign, but now serves to affirm the presence of a community, not just disease prevalence. Using hashtags in post captions literally links users into larger archives of accounts and users. The importance of these anchoring gestures is evident as a trope extends beyond hashtag functionality, including physical signage like @emlwy and @endospoon or part of a username like @the1in10woman. The hashtag serves a similar purpose to the memes that Gomez-Polledo discusses on Tumblr by creating an ecosystem of recognition. But on Instagram, these gestures are just one part of the narrative and remain integrated into personal disclosure and quotidian experience. The hashtags are something regularly deployed to ensure the coordination of disparate illness enactments emerging on an everyday basis through the accounts.

Entanglement: Intra-active Illness on Instagram

In the last examples, in which Instagrammatic hashtags have literally migrated offline and are held by users before being photographically captured and then reintroduced online, helps bring us to entanglement. Entanglement emphasizes how enactments are not just discursive or conceptual, but also deeply physiological. Additionally, it stresses the inextricably intra-active, bidirectional movement between online and offline life. Apparently, offline enactments such as the laparoscopic image are not just brought online; online enactments and forms of coordination also become a fundamental part of living with endometriosis offline. Entanglement's emphatic refusal to draw clear lines between human and nonhuman agents can help flesh out our understanding of these social media narrative structures. In particular, it offers an entryway to engage with the ways in which online and offline life are so interwoven in the narration and basic constitution of illness that they cannot be separated. A recent interview study by Maslen and Lupton (2020) with individuals experiencing chronic illness underscored the complex ways the divide between online/offline disintegrates in the understanding and management of chronic illness. They suggest that their interviews, "demonstrate the complexities of entanglements between human sensory embodied experiences, face-to-face encounters with other people and digitally-mediated experiences and social networks in configuring and enacting lay expertise and self-management of chronic health condition" (1651). As they suggest, the ways illness enactments cross online and offline spaces are difficult to account for without also discarding the paradigm of digital dualism in favor of an alternative model. Distinguishing between what is "nature" and what is "culture," what is "illness" and what is "Instagram" is harder to pull apart than it might at first seem.

Entanglement, as forwarded by Barad (2007), has roots in quantum physics and wide theoretical applicability in a number of fields. Much like enactment, entanglement is fundamentally concerned with multiplicity and the processes by which phenomena are continuously coming into being. Barad emphasizes that not only phenomena like illness are always in process and being done, but that "phenomena are the ontological inseparability of intra-acting agencies" (206). Drawing on notions of realism and measurement embedded in Bohr's atomic model, she stresses that reality is co-constituted by the intra-action of various actors at every moment. In particular, a measurement apparatus does not apprehend separate phenomena that exist in an independent "real world" but is inherently part of those phenomena. In one of her few medical examples, Barad argues that ultrasound "does not peer innocently into the body—it helps produce and is part of the body it images." Social media platforms, the cameras that take posted pictures, and a whole other constellation of technologies involved in this form of media usage are like the ultrasound—not producing a record of offline embodiment and illness experiences, but instead helping produce the ill body itself.

As suggested above, the "1 in 10 selfie" genre of post is one clear example of this entanglement. In this model a digital native construction, the "#1in10," becomes physically conjoined with bodies outside of the platforms. However, this migration offline is primarily driven by the intention to photograph a scene and bring it online. It creates a complex feedback loop that shows how online and offline life continually co-constitute one another. Flow.days's account as a whole is structured in ways that magnify online/offline entanglement even further, illustrating how the social mediated "measurement" of reality is deeply co-constitutive of that reality.[7] Instead of just occasionally blurring the line between reality and Instagram as intermittent #1in10 signs do, flow.days's account hinges on its mixing of self-authored textual posts and pictures of herself holding printed out cards in the style of Instagram squares, using the same font and form as the Instagram posts directly adjacent to them. The only photographs of the individual behind the account are the ones in which she is holding the signs. In other words, her self-portraits are simultaneously portraits of her Instagram account. Discourse structures and Instagrammatic aesthetics become tangible objects, but only as part of a process in which these objects are intended to re-enter virtual narrative spaces. The intra-active relationship between offline enactments and online posts in the constitution of the illness narrative is incredibly clear here, pointing to the way in which envisioning endometriosis offline has become impossible to conceive of without the digital worlds in which the body is inextricably entangled.

Entanglement is particularly evident in #thisisendometriosis challenge posts. This "challenge" emerged out of Georgie Wileman's 2018 art exhibition called "This is Endometriosis," which included various portraits of individuals struggling with the illness.[8] A striking image was a close-up of an abdomen where scars from various laparoscopic surgeries were dated and connected in dark marker. The photograph quickly spread through Instagram endometriosis communities as users made their own abdominal endometriosis "maps" and took pictures of them.[9] The premise of this post itself is only possible because of the physical incisions and the medical conventions, machines, and doctors behind such incisions in the first place. However, a social media-prompted mode of reading those incisions leads individuals to physically mark their own bodies and configure these scars into a particular structure. Furthermore, this activity is not only inspired by Instagram but entangled with it in primarily being done to photograph for a post. Still, more than just bringing the body online, social media tropes and the promise of socially mediated sharing generates a new narrative that is deeply embodied offline in its own right. The act of drawing and labeling creates a story embedded in the body that mobilizes

[7] https://www.instagram.com/flow.days/

[8] See https://www.georgiewileman.com/this-is-endometriosis-1/a71eq434i0pxwvwb7xb6rqalgwp4mc

[9] For more on this campaign and the experience of crip time through Instagram enactments, see my chapter "Chronic Constellations" in the *Routledge Handbook of Media and Health* (2023).

permanent scars into a kind of circular, contained timeline that recontextualizes these incisional traces. In this case, the mutual embeddedness of body and Instagram is so profoundly interwoven that it becomes impossible to demarcate where one ends and the other begins. Blended semiotic structures of numbers, lines, and scars that are derived from both laparoscopic and Instagrammatic modes of envisioning endometriosis are drawn on the material canvas of the chronically ill body in order to surface invisible illness in online spaces.

We can go one step further. Digital culture not only is entangled with conscious user experience and self-narration but becomes part of their organs and cells as well. Psyche and soma, mind and body, intra-act along with online and offline culture. In feminist biologist Wilson's phrasing: "cultural habits become obligated to biology and biology becomes obligated to the psyche" (2004, 22). Illness enactments include psychic practices of story-making and the artistic adoption of Instagrammatic aesthetics not as a distant layer of interpretation but as a fundamental part of the body's matter.

@endospoon's account can help underscore the point that digital life and online tropes do not just co-constitute the idea of illness or how individuals psychically map their own bodies but are intra-actively part of the body at a biological level. This account is primarily composed of beautiful food portraits and recipes, part of a popular canon of healthy living, food, and recipe communities that flourish on Instagram. While such may at first appear to exist in spite of or in addition to her illness and pain, the idea of entanglement helps us see how they are something that both emerges out of the physical body (a means of care and treatment) and helps constitute the body (by determining how it is fueled). Her account bio explains that she is "fighting endometriosis pain with a healthy diet." This fight is not separable from illness or pain, but a key feature of its situated enactment in her body and psyche. Yet, the meals she shares and eats are conditioned by a culture that is fundamentally driven by Instagrammability. Certain foods do not photograph well, especially in this minimalist style. Instagrammatic style therefore alters what a "healthy diet" and what "fighting endometriosis" are by circumscribing what they can look like. As she ingests this food and circulates recipes that her followers can replicate, digital cultures are literally becoming part of her and her readers' bodies.

Even the username, @endospoon joins important facets of posting practices into a single new term can be seen as a kind of entangled Haraway-esque portmanteau: "endo" referring to the endometriosis diagnosis through its social media shorthand; "spoon" capturing both the emphasis on food and eating as well as the social media colloquialism of "spoonie," which is used to refer to chronic illness communities and individuals with chronic illness. In this way, much like natureculture, "endospoon" implicitly challenges boundaries between the biological and the cultural, a blurring that defines the account as a whole and the modes of accounting it relies on.[10] Within the socially mediated illness story, signification and sustenance are impossible to disentangle.

Beyond Remediation

Drawing on premises of feminist technoscience, this chapter has argued that Instagrammatic illness narratives are founded on everyday enactments that entangle the corporeal and the cultural, the sensible and the semiotic. It offers tools to grapple with these stories and practices of storying on their own networked, knotted terms as opposed to constraining ourselves to those that emerged out of earlier work and different mediascapes. It can push researchers to move past the idea of "remediation" as a key to social media narrative scholarship that limits research to questions of comparison and updating. Just as Chun (2016) argues that digital culture is itself governed by a paradigm of "updating to remain the same" scholarship on online narrative runs the risk of petrification in the past if it remains tethered to the logic of the update instead of opening space for alternative modes of theorization. Social media accounts frequently, in and of themselves become modes of accounting for one's illness and illness experience as opposed to simply the latest platforms for telling the same story that could have been communicated through another medium.

While health humanities scholarship has done powerful, invaluable work thus far critiquing the lines between body and discourse, language and illness, digital life requires an approach that even more aggressively focalizes these concerns. The twenty-first century demands that we consider the dynamic, ever-changing communications technologies and virtual environments that, today, continually shape and reshape, define and redefine what a body is. And feminist technoscience—as a field that is frequently on the cutting edge of theorizing this changing, shifting, hybrid

[10] "Spoon theory" was developed by Christine Miserandino in a 2013 blog post as a way of explaining the challenges of everyday life with chronic illness and has been widely adopted online.

body—can push us forward in understanding the dynamic, entangled social media spaces where illness and embodiment are envisioned and enacted every day.

Bibliography

Arduser, Lora. "Remediating Diagnosis: A Familiar Narrative Form or Emerging Digital Genre?." *Emerging Genres in New Media Environments,* edited by Carolyn Miller and Ashley Kelley, Palgrave Macmillan, 2017, pp. 63–78.

Ballweg, Mary Lou. "Impact of Endometriosis on Women's Health: Comparative Historical Data Show that the Earlier the Onset, the More Severe the Disease." *Best Practice & Research Clinical Obstetrics & Gynaecology*, vol. 18, no. 2, 2004, pp. 201–218.

Barad, Karen. *Meeting the Universe Halfway: Quantum Physics and the Entanglement of Matter and Meaning*. Duke UP, 2007.

Bolter, Jay David and Richard Grusin. *Remediation: Understanding New Media.* MIT Press, 2000.

Chun, Wendy Hui Kyong. *Updating to Remain the Same: Habitual New Media.* MIT Press, 2016.

Culley, Lorraine, et al. "The Social and Psychological Impact of Endometriosis on Women's Lives: A Critical Narrative Review." *Human Reproduction Update*, vol. 19, no. 6, 2013, pp. 625–639.

Denny, Elaine. "Women's Experience of Endometriosis." *Journal of Advanced Nursing*, vol. 46, no. 6, 2004, pp. 641–648.

Fausto-Sterling, Anne. "The Bare Bones of Sex: Part 1—Sex and Gender." *Signs: Journal of Women in Culture and Society,* vol. 30, no. 2, 2005, pp. 1491–1527.

Frank, Arthur W. *The Wounded Storyteller: Body, Illness, and Ethics.* 2nd ed., U of Chicago P, 2013.

Gonzalez-Polledo, Elena. "Chronic Media Worlds: Social Media and the Problem of Pain Communication on Tumblr." *Social Media+ Society,* vol. 2, no. 1, 2016, 2056305116628887.

Gonzalez-Polledo, Elena, and Jen Tarr. "The Thing about Pain: The Remaking of Illness Narratives in Chronic Pain Expressions on Social Media." *New Media & Society,* vol. 18, no. 8, 2016, pp. 1455–1472.

Greene, Amanda K. "Chronic Constellations: Instagrammatic Aesthetics and Crip Time." *Routledge Handbook of Health and Media*, edited by Lester D. Friedman & Therese Jones. Routledge, 2023.

Han, Jofen, and Jo Wiley. "Digital Illness Narratives: A New Form of Health Communication." *Transactions of the International Conference on Health Information Technology Advancement,* vol. 2, no. 1, 2013, pp. 47–52. http://scholarworks.wmich.edu/ichita_transactions/18.

Haraway, Donna. *The Companion Species Manifesto: Dogs, People, and Significant Otherness.* Vol. 1. Prickly Paradigm Press, 2003.

Hummelshoj, Lone. "Adhesions," 2018, Endometriosis.org, http://endometriosis.org/endometriosis/adhesions/

Jones, Cara E. "The Pain of Endo Existence: Toward a Feminist Disability Studies Reading of Endometriosis." *Hypatia,* vol. 31, no. 3, 2016, pp. 554–571.

Jurgenson, Nathan. "The IRL Fetish." *The New Inquiry.* https://thenewinquiry.com/the-irlfetish/. June 28, 2012.

Kleinman, Arthur. *The Illness Narratives: Suffering, Healing, and the Human Condition.* Basic Books, 1988.

Markovic, Milica et al. "Endurance and Contest: Women's Narratives of Endometriosis." *Health,* vol. 12, no. 3, 2008, pp. 349–367.

Maslen, Sarah, and Deborah Lupton. "Enacting Chronic Illness with and through Digital Media: A Feminist New Materialist Approach." *Information, Communication & Society,* vol. 23, no. 11, 2020, pp. 1640–1654.

Melander, Ida. "Multimodal Illness Narratives on Instagram: Sharing the Experience of Endometriosis." *DIEGESIS: Interdisciplinary E-Journal for Narrative Research,* vol. 8, no. 2, 2019, pp. 68–90. https://www.diegesis.uni-wuppertal.de/index.php/diegesis/article/download/358/566

Miserandino, Christine. "The Spoon Theory." www.butyoudontlooksick.com, 2013.

Mol, Annemarie. *The Body Multiple: Ontology in Medical Practice.* Duke UP, 2002.

Norman, Abby. *Ask me about my uterus: A quest to make doctors believe in women's pain.* Bold Type Books, 2018.

Porpora, Maria Grazia, et al. "Correlation between Endometriosis and Pelvic Pain." *The Journal of the American Association of Gynecologic Laparoscopists,* vol. 6, no. 4, 1999, pp. 429–434.

Ressler, Pamela Katz, et al. "Communicating the Experience of Chronic Pain and Illness through Blogging." *Journal of Medical Internet Research,* vol. 14, no. 5, 2012, e2002.

Rideout, Victoria, and Susannah Fox. *Digital Health Practices, Social Media Use, and Mental Well-Being Among Teens and Young Adults in the U.S. Hopelab and Well Being Trust.* assets.hopelab.org/wp-content/uploads/2020/08/a-national-survey-by-hopelab-and-well-being-trust-2018.pdf. 2018.

Whelan, Emma. "Putting Pain to Paper: Endometriosis and the Documentation of Suffering." *Health,* vol. 7, no. 4, 2003, pp. 463–482.

Wilson, Elizabeth A. *Psychosomatic: Feminism and the Neurological Body.* Duke UP, 2004.

Narrating Anorexia in Graphic Novels: A Body-Space Analysis

Barbara Grüning

Introduction

This chapter examines the representation of embodiment in fictional and autobiographical graphic narratives about anorexia to show how the so-called anorexic body is not just a surface bearing specific meanings but also a vector of knowledge. For this purpose, I first outline the main discourses on anorexia circulating in the transnational public sphere and in some national public spheres (US, Canada, and countries in Western Europe) carried out by media, institutional actors, and scholars. I will then argue that, even though they depart from different epistemological and moral

B. Grüning (✉)
University of Milan-Bicocca, Milan, Italy
e-mail: barbara.gruning@unimib.it

J. Cressman et al. (eds.), *Envisioning Embodiment in the Health Humanities*, Sustainable Development Goals Series,
https://doi.org/10.1007/978-3-031-49807-7_6

positions, these discourses share a similar iconography,[1] mostly based on timeless images of skinny bodies. As a second step, I look at comics as a medium and its storytelling opportunities that depend on both its "specific material properties" and its social meanings and uses in specific historical contexts (cf. El Refaie 2012: 20). I therefore illustrate how the graphic representation of mental and physical diseases has a long history that has changed over time, in particular with the emergence of the autobiographical genre in the 1970s.

Finally, I analyze eleven graphic narratives which came out during the last twenty years, covering four linguistic areas (English, German, French and Italian) and eight countries (England, United States, Canada, Germany, Austria, Switzerland, France and Italy). The geographic-linguistic dimension is certainly important for understanding the cultural background of the stories and detecting the cultural form of comics or the comics genre in a country. So, for example, the German and Swiss fictional graphic narratives on anorexia are conditioned by a general understanding of comics as a "pedagogical tool" for educating children and teenagers, whereas in France more attention is paid to aesthetic criteria. Due to space constraints and the limited number of graphic novels analyzed, I examine these aspects only marginally. I will instead focus more attention on some crucial, distinctive elements of fictional and autobiographic graphic narratives,[2] such as the different ways in which anorexic subjects are spatialized and temporalized in the stories and the representations of their bodies and bodily practices, which will be the basis for comparison.

[1] The definition used to categorize anorexia are epistemologically and morally not neutral. While anorexia is usually framed through the medical concept of "eating disorder" I adopt here the perspective of people recovering from anorexia, which prefer to define it as "illness", as it emerged from my ongoing investigation of recovery online communities.

[2] The question about the dividing line between fictional and autobiographical narratives has been long discussed (cf. Chaney 2011). Due to space, I will not address the question here. In the chapter I use the term "autobiographical" to indicate that the story narrates episodes and sensations experienced by the author. In this regard, it is not so much a matter of "resemblance with real life" than more of "proximity to discourses of truth and identity" (Gilmore 2001: 3).

The Iconization of Skinny Bodies

Public interest in anorexia and other illnesses related to eating behaviors has often focused on the negative influence on girls and young women coming from widespread cultural models in advertising, the fashion world, and the "star-system" (cf. Malson and Burns 2009).[3] More recently, such public discussion has been extended to also include the phenomenon of "pro-ana" chats and YouTube videos that promote and disseminate an anorexic ethos and lifestyle. The fact that girls and young women have decided to show and perform their skinny bodies (cf. Traue and Schünzel 2014) has aroused opposing "moral" and "epistemic" stances. Within this debate, institutional and media actors, playing the role of "moral entrepreneurs" (Becker 1963), complain about the risks that social media entail for young people. Hence, while "digital anorexics" receive criticism, they are also depicted as unaware of the effects that their curated body images and claims regarding drastic ways of losing weight may have on other girls and young women.

Conversely, many postmodern and post-structuralist feminist scholars consider digital narratives on anorexia as expressions of a subjectivization process. We can pinpoint two steps of their interpretations. First, following a social constructionist perspective, they consider "pro-ana" websites as symptomatic of women's ability to construct an identity independent from a "male gaze" that forces women into a passive role. Second, "pro-ana" digital narratives are counter-narratives that aim at contrasting the categorization of self-starvation as "mental disorder" (Day and Keys 2008; Schott et al. 2016). In short, "pro-ana" websites would counter the normative understanding of the healthy body as proposed, in particular, by institutional and medical actors, as well as a dominant understanding of the female body as a sexualized object. Nevertheless, this interpretative framework of anorexia neglects three crucial aspects of anorexia narratives in social media.

First, social platforms such as YouTube, Tik Tok and Instagram are also used to develop *recovery narratives* (Holmes 2017) based on everyday attempts to heal from this illness. *Second*, social media presents structural constraints that influence how anorexic identities are built and perceived, favoring a specific typification of both these narratives and individuals

[3] Although anorexia and bulimia are not exclusively female phenomena, women represent most of the individuals affected by these illnesses, so the chapter will only refer to them.

suffering from anorexia. While women with anorexia more or less constantly present their everyday life experiences and emotions, the visual organization of social media platforms favors a hasty, casual consumption of textual and audiovisual contents, especially among those who outside recovery or pro-ana communities, or who lack direct experience of the illness. This manner of consumption brings readers to look at the last stories published as detached from ongoing self-narratives (and often without distinguishing these people individually); this way of reading also emphasizes features that may reinforce a common sense of anorexia or "anorexic women" (on the relationship between perception structure and digital media, see: Ignatov 2009; Shaw 2017; Cambre and Lavrence 2019).[4] *Third*, scientific discourses that specifically examine bodies like texts will tend both to isolate them from both the environment where they act (e.g., in the videos) and to neglect more metaphorical and/or indirect forms of expressing a person's *relationship with anorexia over time* rather than merely showing their protruding bones.

In this way, scientific accounts of anorexia risk approaching a common understanding of anorexia, just as the temporal and spatial structure of digital narratives are understood as related to the Therefore, narratives of the concrete experiences of the women who *live with anorexia* are often overlooked as is the idea that women with anorexia experience their illnesses independently from the narrative forms they use to relate their experiences. These circumstances strengthen a social construction of labels (cf. Gilman 1988: 4) and prototypical representations of "anorexic subjects".[5]

When approaching anorexic experiences from a temporal perspective, Darmon (2003) discusses an "anorexic career." An anorexic career generally begins with a diet and often ends with hospitalization. From an interactionist viewpoint (cf. Becker 1963), an anorexic career also typically involves the transformation of the personal identity of women, first into deviant subjects, insofar as their non-conforming acts (starving, throwing up, etc.) are discovered by others, and eventually into patients who occupy an objectified position under the control of medical experts. However,

[4] This aspect has emerged especially clearly by dealing with this topic during my classes in the last four years.

[5] With respect to the issue of how cognitive schemas are embodied and acted through the interaction between human agents and their socio-cultural environment see in particular: Di Maggio (1997), Cerulo (2014), Ignatow (2007), Lizardo (2017).

there are two aspects which Darmon has not fully explored. The first is that, after physically healing, women may retain a distorted perception of their body and relationship with food. The second is that, from a phenomenological viewpoint, women change their entire way of perceiving themselves and the world through their experience of anorexia. Thus, women with anorexia change not only the perception of their bodies, but also the perception of their "social environment" and the position they occupy within it (cf. Löw 2008). This complex transformation of the perceptive disposition creates what Darmon defines as an *anorexic habitus*.

Following Bourdieu's (1980) understanding of habitus, with *anorexic habitus* we intend a set of specific dispositions that women with anorexia develop. The repetition of practices oriented toward losing weight leads to their embodying a specific elitist ethos, the belief that being skinny is proof of being successful and pure (cf. Darmon 2003). This ethos initially gives them the power to continue dieting and throwing up, until these practices are naturalized as part of a taken-for-granted routine. In this manner, their ways of perceiving, thinking about and experiencing themselves and the world is unconsciously modified. The development of these dispositions is also conditioned by the position individuals occupy in society and the social situations they encounter. In this regard, the body is not only a surface where specific meanings are inscribed to forge a specific "anorexic identity", but also a "vector of knowledge" (Wacquant 2000) of the external world used to orient oneself. Identity is then shaped through bodily experiences and signified through the ways that individuals perceive their relationship with the life-world. This interconnection between the anorexic body and the life-world in terms of bodily practices and experiences makes it possible to remodel the concept of identity as a narrative identity (cf. Ricoeur 1988). Narrative identities are here understood as presenting a specific temporal structure which results from the ways of interpreting and interlacing, at a given moment, the various strata of experiences made through the body in different sociocultural contexts (cf. Gugutzer 2002).

Narrative identities are objectified in a medium, and thus are also shaped by the material affordances and social meanings the medium possesses in a given historical context. As El Refaie points out, "each medium emphasizes and de-emphasizes particular aspects of our sensorimotor experience" (2019: 14). I will explore how comics featuring anorexic life stories communicate specific emotions, images, and abstract concepts through their specific ways of *spatializing time*.

Graphic Narratives and Life Stories

Narratives on mental and physical illness have existed throughout the history of comics, reflecting "the changing perception of medicine in society, from the blind faith in the heroic march of medicine of the first part of the twentieth century to the fractured enchantment of the postmodern years" (Williams 2014: 82). In the mid-1970s, the emergence of the autobiographical genre in underground comics marked a meaningful turning point in the representation of mental and physical disturbances. Since the 1990s, with the legitimation of the graphic novel, the autobiographical genre has not only gained prestige, but also taken on a more innovative character, offering "potential new ways of conceptualizing the self" (El Refaie 2012: 19; cf. Kunka 2018).

It is useful to separate features specific to the autobiographical genre from those that more widely characterize the comics medium, even if they have been exploited in the autobiographical genre. Considering these features separately highlights a nonreflective way of absorbing the dominant topics (and sometimes stereotypes) related to anorexia in non-autobiographical comics. Two main features are peculiar to the autobiographical genre. First, like (non-visual) diaries and journals, autobiographical comics are often handmade, which "underscore[s] the subjective positionality of the author" and includes a "subjective mark" of the "body" (Chute 2010: 12). In these cases, the visual-textual narratives may emphasize the subjective marks through pictorial representation, providing the readers with privileged access to the authors' experiences of their life-worlds while suffering from anorexia and their remembered feelings and state of mind. On the other hand, the material cultural support represented by comics allows the authors to make their experience collective.

Second, autobiographical comics provide the possibility for authors to represent their own "physical identity in ways that reflect their own innermost sense of self, often by using a range of symbolic elements and rhetorical tropes to add further layers of meaning to their self-portraits" (cf. El Refaie 2012: 51). The representation of oneself may be reinforced by metaphors, which in comics are composed in three dimensions: the pictorial, which concerns reference to images of concrete objects and scenes; the spatial, which concerns "the position of, and distance between elements in the story, and their relative size, arrangement, and orientation on the page"; and the stylistic, which regards "visual features such as color, form, level of detail, quality of line, and/or visible traces of the means of production" (El Refaie 2019: 16).

Metaphors are particularly powerful in graphic narratives of illness (ibid.: 14). The differences in their uses depend on the ways a specific illness disrupts the equilibrium between the mind, body, and world. Nevertheless, metaphors do not only occur in the autobiographical genre. As noted above, the fact that they are little used in fictional graphic narratives on anorexia is, however, indicative of a low capacity for grasping the feelings of anorexic individuals.

A further feature of comics language, which has flourished thanks to graphic novels, concerns the visualization of memory processes. According to MacCurdy (2007), since images in comics appear in fragments, they are particularly suitable for showing traumatic memory. As a result, graphic narratives may highlight how the attempt to organize life experiences and give them a "meaning" does not result in coherent identities but in hybrid subjectivities. With respect to our topic, however, this feature has been observed only in autobiographical graphic narratives concerning anorexia.

Finally, the meaningful feature of comics language concerns the syntactical operation of representing "time as space" (Chute 2010: 7). Graphic narratives may spatialize different temporal structures in the same space, preventing an unequivocal and linear understanding of the narrated stories. As we will see, in autobiographical narratives on anorexia, this feature has been actualized, for example, by creating palimpsests of past and present events together in the same page or panel, as well as past and present self-portraits of the authors (Chute 2006; cf. El Refaie 2012). More generally, this syntactical operation has been exploited in autobiographical narratives to give expression to the subjective experience of time of the authors' living with anorexia, whereas in fictional graphic narratives on anorexia stories are spatialized in a standard way to build a linear, chronological life story.

In comics, however, space is not only functional to the organization of the temporal dimension of the story. In this regard, we can consider three further interlaced features that can be used as guidelines for the following analysis. The first concerns how physical and social spaces inhabited by anorexic women (i.e., home, school, hospital) are drawn. It is worth noting whether and how the spatial representation changes over the course of the life story, as well as how the positioning of the anorexic body changes in conjunction with the development of an anorexic habitus. The second concerns the interplay between texts and pictures in panels and frames.

The point is not only who talks and what is said, but how thoughts, dialogues, and emotions are spatialized and related to the anorexic body. This means considering whether the interplay between the text, pictures, and other features creates contrasting cognitive and narrative structures or a unified cognitive and narrative structure. Finally, the third level concerns whether and how the interiority of anorexic individuals, as well as their physical and mental illness, are spatialized and materialized.

Analysis of Graphic Narratives on Anorexia

I now provide a deeper insight into the fictional and autobiographical graphic narratives on anorexia, focusing on the general spatial-temporal narrative structure; the thematic frame; the representation of bodies and bodily experiences and, not least, the way the body, mind and life world nexus are represented.

Fictional Accounts

The five fictional graphic narratives on anorexia I consider (*Lucille* 2006; *Durch Dick und Dünn* 2006; *La Chair de l'Araigné* 2010; *41,3 Magersucht?* 2011; *Il Vuoto Intorno a Sandra* 2017) all present sequential time-space structures that reconstruct a linear chronological order from the onset of anorexia to the healing process, so that anorexia is expressed as a "closed" experience.

This sequential temporal structure impacts the ways of representing the subjectivization processes of the protagonists, for which anorexia is almost meant as a stage of identity experiment in their lives, characteristic of youth. In particular, the German, Swiss and Italian graphic novels (*41,2 Magersucht?*; *Durch Dick und Dünn*; *Il Vuoto Intorno a Sandra*) create an explicit nexus between the onset of anorexia and the sense of unease they develop by comparing themselves with "cooler" friends. The two French graphic novels, which represent anorexia either as a form of existential crisis (*Lucille*) or existential lifestyle (*La Chair de l'Araigné*), put more stress on difficult relationships with parents, either in terms of absence (*Lucille*) or conflicts (*La Chair de l'Araigné*). In any case, all five graphic novels describe eating disorders as deriving from the desire or refusal to fulfill specific social expectations, which are embodied by "specific others" (Mead 1942). Furthermore, in the German and Swiss graphic novels, the healing process is aided by medical experts (in Mead's terms, by "generalized others" [1934]) who allow the young protagonists to correctly continue their socialization process.

The stories are spatially structured to create a regular rhythm, alternating comic panels that function to develop the plot with freeze-images, which highlight typified features of anorexic bodies and practices, such as looking in the mirror to perceive a deformed image of their own body, partaking in physical exercise, or weighing themselves. In the two French graphic novels, we also find some flashbacks to the protagonists' childhoods, which show, more or less, how the conscious decision to transform their bodies derives from a deep discontent regarding their self-image. Thus, beyond the identification of social causes that have favored the onset of anorexia, we find a clear definition of anorexia as a disorder primarily bound to physical appearance. As a result, the body is only seen as an object of perception and not as a "vector of knowledge" through which anorexic subjects form the perception of themselves in relation to the spatial environment. Thus, little attention is paid to the represented space, which seems to have two main uses. In the German and Swiss graphic novels, the spatial environment plays only a deictic role to identify specific places (home, school, hospital, etc.) that represent a normative bourgeois society. In the Italian and French graphic novels, the spatial environment also performs a symbolic function in depicting specific cultural milieux and lifestyles. Examples include the desolation of Sandra's home in a peripheral urban area (Fig. 1) and a bohemian flat in *La Chair de l'Araigné*, which stresses the idea anorexia is a free choice of the protagonists and corresponding to the desire of embracing anorexia as a specific lifestyle.

Finally, the text-image interplay in these graphic narratives complies with its standard use. The verbal elements through which opinions, emotions, thoughts, and dialogues are expressed follow a classical presentation within speech balloons. In the French and Italian graphic novels some panels without balloons and text create a pause for reflection in the storytelling, stressing a protagonist's specific mood, but has a more deictic than existential nature. As a result, in the fictional graphic novels there are two main ways of narrating anorexia and the anorexic body. Anorexic bodies are either verbally thematized (especially in the German and Swiss educational graphic novels, which reproduce a medical viewpoint), or they are figuratively symbolized in a mimetic way by condensing some specific features which make it easy to identify "anorexic individuals" as "social types". The interiorization process of the illness, which is its very form of embodiment, is therefore blurred.

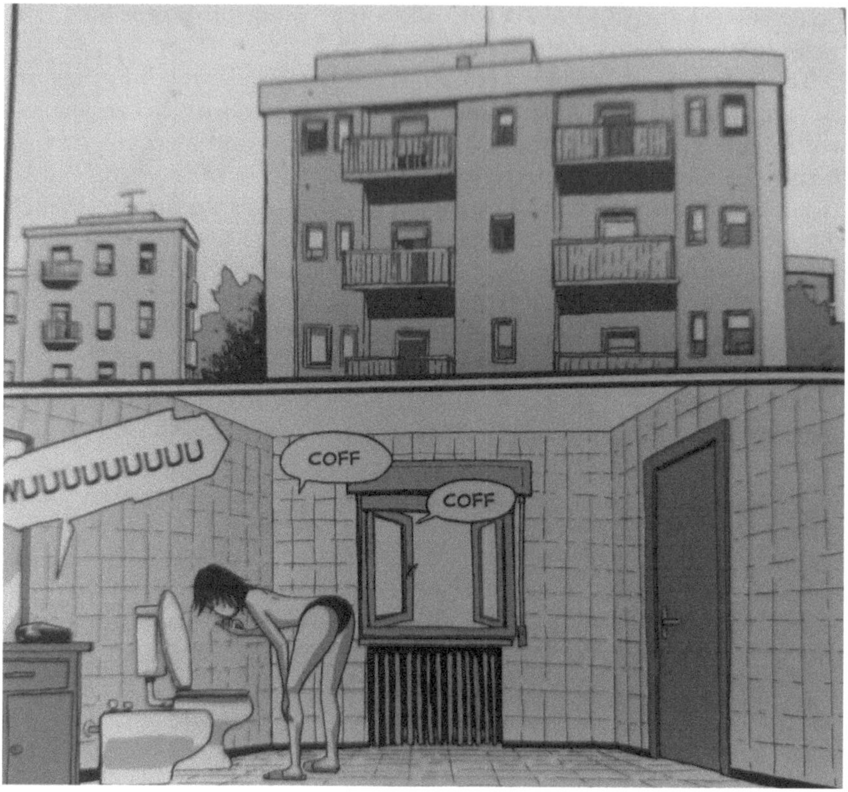

Fig. 1 Panel of the graphic novel *Il Vuoto Intorno a Sandra*

Autobiographical Texts

The six autobiographical graphic narratives in this sample (*Inside Out* 2007; *Lighter than My Shadow* 2013; *Tyranny* 2009; *Ink in Water* 2017; *Blad* 2018; *Cheese* 2019) present a more complex space-time structure than fictional graphic narratives, providing more storytelling opportunities and narrative strategies. The narrated time may be either longer than the anorexic phase, crossing multiple biographical crises, before, during, and after anorexia, up to and including the moment of their autobiographical writing (*Inside Out*; *Lighter than My Shadow*; *Tyranny*; *Ink in Water*), or it ends with a sort of blackout, suggesting the anorexic phase has not concluded (*Blad*), or the narrative may sink into a specific phase of the anorexic experience, leaving its temporal contour shaded (*Cheese*). In each case, the graphic narratives do not present a clear ending of the illness. In addition, those who narrate the post-anorexia phase bring out the daily struggle of the protagonists to come to terms with their anorexic habitus, which continues to survive after the more acute phase of self-starvation, and thus the continuous struggle to give sense to the different fragments of the self they have collected over time.

To highlight the difficulty of living with anorexia and overcoming it, autobiographical graphic narratives exploit the interplay between text and image in innovative ways. Not rarely, blank or black pages, sometimes containing scribbled words, alternate with either outsized images of the torn anorexic body, where it seems no words may be uttered (see, in particular, *Lighter than My shadow*, *Ink in Water* and *Cheese*), or with deformed fragments of the body (see especially *Blad*).

Thus, what occurs in these moments is a short circuit between words and images, between what might be said but which is impossible to say, and between what might be seen but which is impossible to see. As a result, not only do life stories gain synesthetic depth, but the storytelling appears discordant, stressing the impossibility of expressing and communicating feelings and thoughts through common verbal forms. Indeed, this split between text and image mirrors the "double life" of anorexic women, the separation between their interior life and what remains of a "normal life," in the rare moments when they are still able to engage in dialogue with other people and to continue their old everyday activities. In other words, the spatial structure of the stories undermines narrative time, creating at the same time a space for the clouding of the protagonist's consciousness so that the individual consciousness is spatially expanded through the eclipse of narrative time.

The spatialization of consciousness also occurs metaphorically through the anthropomorphization of anorexia, even if it takes rather the form of monsters. What is noteworthy is that anthropomorphized anorexia or bulimia not only occupies the mind and the body of the protagonists, but also invades their "life-world" until it constitutes their primary and almost exclusive social relationship. A further narrative device is the failing of physical coordinates in both the spatial environment and structure, as in *Inside Out* and *Tyranny*. The lack of physical coordinates expresses, at the same time, the lack of social and relational coordinates for the anorexic subject, as she is outside of every sort of social and material space.

In these autobiographical graphic narratives, making sense of one's life is not so much a question of rationally and chronologically organizing the different negative and positive events which the protagonists have lived before, during, and after anorexia. Instead, it is a question of finding a way of expressing and communicating their own perceptions and feelings towards their bodies, others, and their life world. This effort requires an ongoing reflection, as memory work not only for understanding what has happened, but also for how to consciously lead their lives in an anorexic habitus. Autobiographical graphic novels finally show a permanent need to train oneself, and learn, to feel normal (*Tyranny*; *Inside Out*; *Ink in Water*; *Lighter than My Shadow*). Thus, differently from fictional graphic novels about anorexia (*Lucille*; *Durch Dick und Dünn*; *La Chair de l'Araigné*; *41,2 Magersucht?*; *Il Vuoto Intorno a Sandra*), they illustrate the impossibility of giving predefined social explanations for the states of mind and feelings of anorexic individuals. At the same time, they also emphasize two understandings of the body that are difficult to grasp in the fictional graphic narratives: on the one hand, the body as an acculturated body (*Körper*) which is discursively constructed through social meanings, and, on the other hand, the body is experienced by its own consciousness (*Leib*) (cf. Knoblauch 2005). By privileging the second dimension over the first, in autobiographical narratives, the representation of the author-protagonist is rarely mimetic. The body is often transfigured in order to mirror their feelings and take distance from their narrated selves. Within the spatial structure, the transfigured body as well as the representation of individual parts of the body of the life stories also open an interpretative space to readers for understanding the complexity of living *with* anorexia, stressing moreover how it is difficult to give any coherent solution to one's own identity and story.

Discussion and Conclusion

Cultural narratives on anorexia conceive of the illness as depending either on external social forces which negatively influence young women, as if they were passive individuals, or on the will of the young women to shape their bodies in order to tackle the dominant categorizations of female bodies that are widespread in society. Within this complex of discourses, independent of the moral and epistemological stance expressed, the focus is almost exclusively on the form and dimension of the female body, whereas little attention is paid to the concrete experiences and feelings of women who live with anorexia. Hence, this chapter has aimed to analyze how fictional and autobiographical graphic narratives deal with the issue, taking into account the storytelling opportunities that the comics medium offers. In this regard, fictional and non-fictional graphic narratives have been compared on the basis of their space-time narrative structure, the interplay between text and image, and the ways of representing the relationship between body, mind and life-world.

In the fictional graphic narratives, the space-time narrative structure is mostly used to chronologically describe the development of the illness and to explain the social causes of anorexia. The transformation of sensorial perception brings only a distorted image of one's own body, without consequences on the ways of perceiving the spatial environment. This is also evident by the standardized use of speech balloons for communicating and expressing feelings and thoughts and by a deictic or, in some cases, a symbolic function that is useful for catching specific social and (sub)cultural milieux of the spatial background. If the disruption of the illness changes the ways of seeing one's own body, it does not undermine the sense of being in the world. In this regard, fictional graphic narratives share a perspective with cultural discourses on anorexia. These narratives represent anorexia experience as something concluded and related to a specific phase of the life, corresponding to adolescence.

Conversely, autobiographical graphic narratives use the space-time narrative structure in innovative ways by creating a sense of spatial and temporal disorientation to which the disorientation in the social world experienced by anorexic women correspond as well. The difficulty of communicating their emotions and thoughts is expressed by the disjunction of text and image which creates two opposite structures of meaning. Whereas in the fictional graphic novels the protagonists appear as bi-dimensional, in the autobiographical graphic narratives the materiality of their pain is communicated by making the interiority of the protagonists visible, and materially disgusting. The relationship between body and mind is so mediated by an anthropomorphized anorexia, which as a deformed being colonizes both and also comes out from the body, that it occupies the spatial environment surrounding the protagonists. Nevertheless, only the anorexic individuals are able to see and feel what is occurring inside and outside of them. As noted earlier, the representation of the author-protagonist is rarely mimetic. Instead, these life stories open an interpretative space to readers for understanding the complexity of living *with* anorexia, stressing the impossibility of presenting a neatly confined narrative.

Bibliography

Becker, Howard S. *Outsiders: Studies in the Sociology of Deviance*. New York: The Free Press of Glencoe, 1963.

Bourdieu, Pierre. *Le sens pratique*. Éditions de Minuit, 1980.

Cambre, Maria-Carolina, and Christine Lavrence. "How Else Would You Take a Photo? #SelfieAmbivalence." *Cultural Sociology*, vol. 13, no. 4, 2019, pp. 503–24.

Cerulo, Karen A. "Continuing the Story: Maximizing the Intersections of Cognitive Science and Sociology." *Sociological Forum* (Randolph, N.J.), vol. 29, no. 4, 2014, pp. 1012–19.

Chaney, Michael A. *Graphic Subjects: Critical Essays on Autobiography and Graphic Novels*. U of Wisconsin P, 2011.

Chute, Hillary L. *Graphic Women: Life Narrative and Contemporary Comics*. Columbia UP, 2010.

———."'The Shadow of a Past Time': History and Graphic Representation in Maus." *Twentieth Century Literature*, vol. 52, no. 2, 2006, pp. 199–230.

Darmon, Muriel. *Devenir anorexique. Une approche sociologique*. Paris: Editions la Decouverte, 2003.

Davis, Lacy J., and Jim Kettner. *Ink in Water: An Illustrated Memoir: Or, How I Kicked Anorexia's Ass and Embraced Body Positivity!* New Harbinger Publications, Inc., 2017.

Day, Katy, and Keys, Tammy. "Starving in Cyberspace: A Discourse of Pro-eating Disorder Websites." *Gender Studies*, vol. 17, no. 1, 2008, pp. 1–15.

Debeurme, Ludovic. *Lucille*. Futuropolis, 2006.

DiMaggio, Paul. "Culture and Cognition." *Annual Review of Sociology*, vol. 23, no. 1, 1997, pp. 263–87.

El Refaie, Elisabeth. *Autobiographical comics. Life Writing in Pictures*. Jackson: University Press of Mississipi, 2012.

———. *Visual Metaphor and Embodiment in Graphic Illness Narratives*. Oxford UP, 2019.

Fairfield, Lesley. *Tyranny*. Tundra Books, 2009.

Gilman, Sander L. *Disease and Representation: Images of Illness from Madness to AIDS*. New York: Cornell, 1988.

Gilmore, Leigh. *The Limits of Autobiography: Trauma and Testimony*. Cornell UP, 2001.

Green, Katie. *Lighter than My Shadow*. Random House, 2013.

Gugutzer, Robert. *Leib, Körper, Identität*. Westdeutscher Verlag, 2002.
Heimgartner, Susanna and Karin Schneider. *Durch Dick und Dünn*. Schulverlag, 2006.
Hofer, Regina. *Blad*. Luftschacht, 2018.
Holmes, Su. "'My Anorexia Story': Girls Constructing Narratives of Identity on YouTube." *Cultural Studies* (London, England), vol. 31, no. 1, 2017, pp. 1–23.
Hubert, and Marie Caillou. *La chair de l'Airaigné*. Éditions Glénat, 2010.
Ignatow, Gabriel. "Theories of Embodied Knowledge: New Directions for Cultural and Cognitive Sociology?" *Journal for the Theory of Social Behaviour*, vol. 37, no. 2, June 2007, pp. 115–35.
———. "Culture and Embodied Cognition: Moral Discourses in Internet Support Groups for Overeaters." *Social Forces*, vol. 88, no. 2, Dec. 2009, pp. 643–69.
Knoblauch, Hubert. "Kulturkörper." *Soziologie des Körpers*. Edited by Markus Schroer, Suhrkamp, 2005, pp. 92–113.
Kunka, Andrew. *Autobiographical Comics*. Bloomsbury Academic, an Imprint of Bloomsbury Publishing Plc, 2018.
Lizardo, Omar. "Improving Cultural Analysis: Considering Personal Culture in Its Declarative and Nondeclarative Modes." *American Sociological Review*, vol. 82, no. 1, Feb. 2017, pp. 88–115.
Löw, Martina. "The Constitution of Space. The Structuration of Spaces through the Simultaneity of Effect and Perception." *European Journal of Social Theory*, vol. 11, no. 1, February 2008, pp. 25–49.
MacCurdy, Marian M. *The Mind's Eye: Image and Memory in Writing about Trauma*. U of Massachusetts P, 2007.
Malson, Helen, and Maree Burns, editors. *Critical Feminist Perspectives on Eating Dis/Orders*. London: Routledge, 2009.
Mead, George Herbert. *Mind, Self and Society*. Chicago: Chicago University Press, 1942.
Ricoeur, Paul. "L'identité narrative." *Esprit*, vol. 7, no. 8, juillet/août 1988, pp. 295–304.
Sabisch, Ingrid. *41,3 kg Magersucht?* Gütersloher Verlagshaus, 2011.
Schott, Nicole D., et al. "Neoliberalism, Pro-Ana/mia Websites, and Pathologizing Women: Using Performance Ethnography to Challenge Psychocentrism." *Studies in Social Justice*, vol. 10, no. 1, 2016, pp. 95–115.
Shaw, Adrienne. "Encoding and Decoding Affordances: Stuart Hall and Interactive Media Technologies." *Media, Culture & Society*, vol. 39, no. 4, 2017, pp. 592–602.
Shivak, Nadia. *Inside Out: Portrait of An Eating Disorder*. Atheneum, 2007.
Traue, Boris and Anja Schünzel. "Visueller Aktivismus und affektive Öffentlichkeiten: Die Inszenierung von Körperwissen in 'Pro Ana' und 'Fat Acceptance' Blogs." *Österreichische Zeitschrift für Soziologie*, vol. 39, no. 1, 2014, pp. 121–142.
Valentini, Fabio. *Il vuoto intorno a Sandra*. Shockdom, 2017.

Wacquant, Loïc. *Body and Soul: Notebooks of an Apprentice Boxer.* Oxford UP, 2000.
Williams, Ian C. M. "Graphic Medicine: The Portrayal of Illness in Underground and Autobiographical Comics." *Medicine, Health and the Arts: Approaches to the Medical Humanities*, edited by Victoria Bates, et al., Routledge, 2014, pp. 64–84.
Zuzu. *Cheese.* Coconino Press 2019.

Rehearsing Grief: Turning to Look at Loss in *Eurydice*

Elizabeth Lanphier

Introduction

As the editors of this collection note, embodied experience is always partial, liminal, and incomplete. Thus the knowledge attained from embodied experience is always from a particular perspective that cannot be fully shared with another. Yet, as the editors also indicate, language is also incomplete and cannot communicate the depth of embodied knowledge that one experiences in and for the self. Live theater uniquely combines embodied experience and language. The playwright conveys a story through words that are intended to be embodied. This story is co-produced with actors interpreting and reciting the lines, directors interpreting and enacting stage directions, teams of set dressers, lighting experts and sound technicians shaping the space in which the play is

E. Lanphier (✉)
Department of Pediatrics, University of Cincinnati College of Medicine, Cincinnati, OH, USA

Ethics Center, Cincinnati Children's Hospital Medical Center, Cincinnati, OH, USA
e-mail: elizabeth.lanphier@cchmc.org

J. Cressman et al. (eds.), *Envisioning Embodiment in the Health Humanities*, Sustainable Development Goals Series,
https://doi.org/10.1007/978-3-031-49807-7_7

performed, and received by an audience also co-producing meaning through their unique embodied experience of watching that particular play in that particular moment. Though any individual production may be staged multiple times per day or week during its run, an individual performance is a uniquely fleeting embodied encounter between performers and audience, never to be repeated exactly the same way again.

This unique form of theatrical embodiment is particularly striking in Sarah Ruhl's play *Eurydice*, which reimagines the Orpheus and Eurydice myth from the point of view of the alive, and then dead, Eurydice. The play does something that neither life, nor many other art forms, cannot: it embodies the experience of *being dead,* and affords the audience an embodied experience of confronting the embodied experiences of dead characters, as well as inanimate objects ("the Stones"), which are performed by human actors.[1] In Ruhl's distinctive theatrical imagination, what is alive and what is dead is not so easy to differentiate. There is no set change to distinguish between the underworld and the "overworld" (land of the living).

From a health humanities perspective, *Eurydice* does something exceptional by inviting empathy not only with those experiencing the death of another or imagining the loss of the self, but by literally sitting with another who is herself dead, yet present to the audience. Thus the play invites the audience to also sit with feelings of grief for the self in our own deaths in an entirely original way thanks to the embodied experience of giving and receiving a story through theater. It is arguably the pain Eurydice experiences in the underworld, once dead, and the pain of her father, who we only encounter as dead in the underworld, that is most empathetically recognizable to the audience, provoking the viewer's sympathy. Ruhl gives the audience access to the pain of one who is no longer living, and invites us to try on and test out experiences of others who are grieving, but also, importantly, ourselves, by imagining an underworld populated by thinking and feeling stones and dead characters.

Theater reviews of *Eurydice* note the play's production of intense emotion in its audience. Critics from the *New York Times* described the play as possibly "the most moving exploration of the theme of loss" in American theater thus far in the twenty-first century. One critic, who is accustomed

[1] There are three characters that collective Ruhl refers to as "the Stones" and which are specifically "Big Stone," "Little Stone," and "Loud Stone." In this chapter I capitalize "Stones" when talking about the characters, but use "stones" without capitalization when talking about stones as inanimate objects, and I follow text in capitalizing or not when I directly quote Ruhl.

to crying at the theater and, so, generally able to anticipate it, found that watching *Eurydice* triggered an altogether different experience: "the tears came with the suddenness of grief" (Al-Shamma 2011, 14). Writing in the *Boston Globe*, Louise Kennedy recounted viewing the play a month after her father's death. While she "had gone through the rituals of mourning," she found it hard to cry. It was watching *Eurydice* that prompted more intense and sustained tears (Al-Shamma 2011, 14).

James Al-Shamma discusses the play's engagement with grief, and particularly its demonstration of the mourning or grieving process mapped by Sigmund Freud, John Archer, and the four stages of grief from John Bowlby, concluding that the play moves through three of the four stages (Al-Shamma 2011, 33). For Al-Shamma, "the process of grieving is abruptly cut off at the conclusion of the play" and "reorganization" or the "recovery from bereavement" is not achieved (Al-Shamma 2011, 36). I am most interested not in the grieving process internal to the play as much as the *staging of* grief: the intersubjectivity of grieving that the play sparks *between* characters, and between the action internal to the play and the audience viewing it. I have written before about the co-construction of meaning between art and viewer (Lanphier 2020), and *Eurydice* enacts a particular kind of co-constructed experience among audience and actor.

In his *Philosophical Investigations*, Ludwig Wittgenstein explores how we could ever truly come to understand the experience of another, and the limitation of both language and imagination, which we shape within our own points of view. In this essay I suggest that while the embodied nature of theater affords a certain horizon of experience and limitation of perspective, it also opens up new channels of experience that can only be accessed through embodiment. For example, Wittgenstein often invokes a stone. He asks, "could one imagine a stone's having consciousness?" (Wittgenstein 2009, §390). Ruhl's play does just that. She creates three characters who are Stones, with consciousness. Wittgenstein offers that "what has a mind, what have pains, to do with a stone? Only what behaves like a human being can one say that it *has* pains" (Wittgenstein 2009, §283).

Ruhl gives the Stones as characters bodies and minds; they have their own language, "the language of stones" (Ruhl 2006, 360), which is also the "language of dead people" (Ruhl 2006, 359). Ruhl creates a theatrical world that asks us to "look at a stone and imagine it having sensations" (Wittgenstein 2009, §284). She opens up something Wittgenstein takes to be inaccessible to us, and to which pain does not typically apply: being dead.[2] The play invites the audience to discover that "[o]ur attitude to what is alive and to what is dead is not the same. All our reactions are different" (Wittgenstein 2009, §284).

Eurydice is both groundbreaking original theater and a thought experiment for the very challenges to imagination Wittgenstein identifies in the *Philosophical Investigations.* Close reading *Eurydice*, especially in its engagement with the uncanny and repetition, shows how theater is specifically suited to do conceptual and emotive work with regards to how an audience physically confronts and considers death and grief. The play generates empathic understanding of grief within a community of participants (the audience) tasked with continually reacting, participating, imagining, and seeing anew.

Allusion, Rehearsal, and a Nod Toward the Uncanny

Eurydice revisits the classical Orpheus and Eurydice myth reimagined from the point of view of Eurydice. The original tale, told by both Virgil and Ovid, centers the perspective of Orpheus, a renowned musician whose wife Eurydice dies soon after their wedding. Orpheus plays music at the gates of Hades to bring her back from the underworld. He is able to return her to the world of the living on the condition he trust she is following him back to the overworld: he cannot look at her until they have left the underworld completely. But he does look back, and she immediately returns to the underworld where she will remain. Ruhl imagines the story from the view and voice of Eurydice: her experience marrying Orpheus, arriving in the underworld, possibly returning to Orpheus and the world of the living, but ultimately not. Ruhl's *Eurydice* is also a father daughter tale: Eurydice is reunited with her dead father in the underworld.[3] Situating the play in ancient myth is an invocation of repetition, the repeating of a familiar story. There is a particular enactive imagination at work in *Eurydice* in which the imagination is something that is actively doing (creating a new artistic work, generating a new perspective) and participatory (through the staging, performance and reception of the

[2] Put differently, Ruhl's "dead" characters are in fact very alive: they move, speak, breath, express, emote. They also feel physical and emotional pain, which is quite different from how we typically think and talk about death as releasing people from physical or emotional pain and suffering.

[3] Ruhl dedicated the play to her own deceased father.

piece of theater).[4] Imagination is dramatic rehearsal,[5] here being quite literally dramatically rehearsed.

The play dramatically rehearses shifts between the worlds of the living and the dead, the animate and inanimate, complicating the borders between both, since embodied, living actors perform both alive and dead characters. The character of Eurydice appears the same whether alive or dead; the three Stones are supposedly inanimate objects personified and performed by three actors, with movement and language. These seemingly strange aspects of the play become familiar within the imaginative world of the theater, forcing the viewer to consider the uncanny, what it means to find the unknown in the familiar, or to be at home in a strange place, just as the familiar story of Orpheus and Eurydice is rendered strange to us by the play itself. Theatrical rehearsal itself flirts with the uncanny. The word begins with the prefix "re" to repeat, and "hercer," French for "harrow." The verb "to harrow" holds dual meanings. Its most literal form describes a farming technique using a harrow, a sharp or spiked edge implement, to plow land. But "harrow" also means to terrify, frighten, or mortify. The uncanny is unsettling, it has the capacity to be harrowing, and it is invoked through its repetition, though slightly askew, of the familiar.

The Familiar Unfamiliar

Eurydice begins with the domestic: Orpheus and Eurydice are in love and engaged.[6] The next scene is their wedding. Eurydice's father left her a letter saying "if I were to give a speech at your wedding I would start with one or two funny jokes, and then I might offer some words of advice." His advice contained seven points, half about mundane household tasks: techniques for cooking fish and toast; keeping dogs as companions; and a reminder to "take care to change the light bulbs" (Ruhl, 343). The shift from the overworld to underworld is a rupture from the ordinary, when

[4] See Richard Moran. "The Expression of Feeling in Imagination." *Philosophical Review* Vol. 103, no. 1 (1994): 75–106.

[5] Again, in the phrase of Moran who talks of the dramatic rehearsal of the imagination (Moran 1994).

[6] While I cannot fully explore this connection in the space of this chapter, I want to draw attention to the ways in which the domesticity of the play connects to Stanley Cavell's notion of ordinary language and the connection of the ordinary and uncanny. See Cavell (1988).

what is home is made unhomely; from the underworld, Eurydice's father is preoccupied by the ordinariness of home.

This shift begins within the letter from Eurydice's father. After his imagined marital speech, he goes on to say: "as for me, this is what it's like being dead. … the atmosphere smells. And there are strange high-pitched noises—like a tea kettle always boiling over. But it doesn't seem to bother anyone. And, for the most part, there is a pleasant atmosphere and you can work and socialize, much like at home" (344). Two similes connect the domestic and the dead: the noise is "*like* a tea kettle" and it is "*much like* at home," yet it is not a tea kettle and it is not home; it is the afterlife. The uncanny is the resemblance to the familiar that is not familiar.

In his essay "The Uncanny," Freud provides an etymology of *heimlich* and *unheimlich*, or canny and uncanny. *Heimlich* is "belonging to the house, not strange, familiar, tame, dear and intimate, homely, etc." (Freud 2003, 126) while its antonym, *unheimlich*, "etymologically corresponds to 'unhomely'" based on this definition of *heimlich*, or "unfamiliar," but these definitions miss the element of fearfulness that unheimlich connotes. Per Freud "the uncanny is that species of frightening that goes back to what was once well known and had long been familiar" and that it is an "intellectual uncertainty" that renders some unfamiliar situations "in which a person was unsure of his way around" uncanny (Freud 2003, 124–125). *Eurydice* performs the uncanny through staging in which everything we visually see is familiar, but both we and the characters are at times unsure of our way around.

In the second movement of the play, Eurydice knows she has died, yet she does not understand that she is in the underworld.[7] Ruhl's stage directions describe: "The Underworld. There is no set change. Strange watery noises. Drip, drip, drip. The movement to the underworld is marked by the entrance of stones" (Ruhl 2006, 357). Ruhl offers no material distinction between the world of the living and the world of the dead; the set is already familiar to the audience (and to Eurydice), but it is rendered strange by the background noises and the addition of what the stage directions appear to describe as inanimate objects, but which are in fact are three characters—actors—playing "stones." In Ruhl's notes on the play she indicates that "the set should allow for fluid transitions from moment

[7] Again, Cavell is useful here, particularly in his distinction between knowing and acknowledging. Eurydice demonstrates the possibility to *know* something without in fact acknowledging it. See Cavell (1969).

to moment—from underworld to overworld and back again" (Ruhl 2006, 332). The imperceptibility of whether we are viewing the world of the living or dead, whether the actors are playing characters alive or dead, contribute to the uncanny. Audience and protagonist share in the "intellectual uncertainty."

Eurydice believes she is on a vacation. She has her traveling attire and suitcase. She encounters her father, already dead in the underworld, and does not recognize him; thinking him a hotel porter, she asks to be taken to her room. Her father responds, half-playing the role of porter, half-assuaging her misconception, saying, "I'm sorry, miss, but there are no rooms here." Eurydice responds with "What? No rooms? Where do people sleep," to which her father replies, "people don't sleep here" (365). Her father plays into her desire for the familiarity and safety of a room, while helping her acknowledge that she is in an entirely different place, one that functions differently than the world of the living.

Eurydice tries to make this strange world familiar by imposing her assumptions onto the space. Her father tries to provide familiarity. When she is "on the verge of tears" according to the stage directions, the Stones in unison tell her "Don't cry! Don't cry!" (Ruhl 2006, 366), and later they say that "being sad is not allowed! Act like a stone" in the face of Eurydice's sadness in the underworld (373). Seeing her sadness, her father asks her to not "be sad. I'll take your luggage to your room," while the Stones shout in chorus "THERE ARE NO ROOMS!" Her father "picks up her luggage. He gives the Stones a dirty look" (Ruhl 2006, 366). The Stones want to maintain the norms of the underworld, without tears, without rooms, without memories, without names, and without the language of the living.[8] The father wants to protect his daughter from this similar yet different world by building her a new "room" as she requested. In a wordless scene that the stage notes describe, "The Father creates a room out of string for Eurydice. He makes four walls and a door out of string. Time passes. It takes time to build a room out of string. Eurydice observes the underworld. There isn't much to observe" (Ruhl 2006, 367).

What is observable about the underworld is its resemblance to the "overworld," matched with the sense that things are slightly askew. The

[8] Playing the role of a Greek chorus, the Stones in unison address the audience after Eurydice arrives to the underworld and opens her mouth to speak but no words come out, explaining "Eurydice wants to speak to you. But she can't speak your language anymore. She talks in the language of dead people now" (359).

"language of dead people" is "a very quiet language," according to the Stones (Ruhl 2006, 359), and though they are presumably speaking this quiet, dead people language, they speak in English. At one point, the Stones invite the audience into a thought experiment: imagine that their language is comprehensible by imagining that we understand Eurydice speaking to us (which, of course, we can): "pretend for a moment that you understand the language of stones … listen to her the way you would listen to your own daughter if she died too young and tried to speak to you across long distances" (Ruhl 2006, 360). We are asked to imagine a language we do not understand, "like potatoes sleeping in the dirt" (Ruhl 2006, 360), a simile so absurd that it requires its own engagement with the imagination to comprehend, in order to re-imagine that we do understand it. This task of imagining Euryicide's experience of being dead and empathizing with her experience is connected to also imagining her death as a loss we personally experience and grieve, like a mourning parent. Thus the audience is invited to both empathize with her and with the experience of losing her.

Wittgenstein claimed we cannot access the pain of a corpse, yet Ruhl's play actively embodies the pain of a dead person. When the Stones ask the audience to imagine Eurydice's experience by imagining mourning her loss, this recalls Wittgenstein's assertion to "not ask yourself: 'How does it work with *me*?'—Ask: 'What do I know about someone else'" (Wittgenstein 1982, Fragment xi §204). Wittgenstein underlines the inter-subjectivity of subjective experience. We can imagine the experience of the other although it is only from our subjective position. *Eurydice* does just that: we consider the experience for another person, but do so by imagining an experience also for ourselves. This is a kind of imagination unique, in some ways, to theater, where the experiences of imagined others are enacted in real time in the presence of an audience attentive to and working alongside the performers, to co-construct the experience and create meaning in the imagined time and place of the performance, that also connects to prior memories, and future imagined experience.

This is, I take it, precisely why so many reviewers recount an intense experience of personal emotion either during, or soon after, watching *Eurydice* on stage. The audience does not merely witness art, they are drawn into the enactive imagination of the play, experiencing alongside the cast and fellow viewers. Tapping into the experience for someone else is what also ignites awareness of the experience for the self: Kennedy's ability to shed tears for her own father that were restrained until she experienced the losses between father and daughter in *Eurydice*, for example. Most interestingly, as a work of theater physically staged by performers and witnessed by an audience, *Eurydice* creates an occasion for the audience to have embodied experiences that are otherwise hard to imagine let alone feel in our bodies, like proximate loss and grief, or even impossible to experience otherwise, like being able to reflect and report on the embodied experience our own (in this case imagined) death and what it is like to be dead.

Stanley Cavell (1988) takes there to be three possible responses to the uncanny and loss, all three of which are demonstrated within *Eurydice*: the display of grief and mourning (by Orpheus); the distraction of loss (or perhaps its denial, the desire to see differently, by Eurydice); and the rebuilding or reconstructing of something new in the face of loss (the string room, which reimagines the space of the underworld, in which there are no rooms). The underworld of *Eurydice* is uncanny, but also reading alongside Wittgenstein, it is like his ancient city, which is a maze of old and new, at once navigable but unfamiliar, in which it is possible to orient, but is disorienting (Wittgenstein 2009, §18). In the underworld, like the ancient city, space can be reimagined, and new structures can be erected, such as the string room.

Al-Shamma discusses *Eurydice*'s depiction of Archer's adaptation of Bowlby's grief process: numbness and disbelief; yearning and searching; disorganization and despair; reorganization and recovery (Al-Shamma 2011, 33) to suggest that the play never achieves the fourth stage of reorganization (36). Yet reorganization need not be narrowly understood as complete recovery. Cavell and Wittgenstein allow for reorganization to be a process of building, rebuilding, or seeing anew—in ways that allow for this to be a transformative process. The play itself rebuilds our understanding of grief itself: in staging grief it moves us through grief's stages. It allows for the development of familiarity with the unfamiliar. That is to say that watching the play makes something relatively unfamiliar to us, like grief (especially if we have yet to encounter it) more familiar or makes unfamiliar something we may already find familiar (grief, again, if we have already encountered it) that we can see anew.

Repetition

Part of how *Eurydice* uniquely plays with the uncanny and grief is through repetition. The play repeats an uncanny version of the myth of Orpheus and Eurydice. And on a meta-level, the play is a piece of theater re-performed night after night, and across various productions. Music is both theme and presence in the play. Orpheus is a musician, and repetition, rehearsal, and motif as part of music is constantly invoked. In the opening scene, foreshadowing much of the action to come, Orpheus tries to teach Eurydice a melody, but her rhythm is off. Orpheus tells her "we'll practice"; practice requires repetition through rehearsal. Their rehearsal that the audience watches on stage is also the embodiment of the repetition of rehearsal that went into the theatrical production the audience is now witnessing. When Orpheus asks Eurydice if she will remember his melody, she emphatically retorts, "Yes! I WILL ALWAYS REMEMBER YOUR MELODY!" (Ruhl 2006, 338). This scene of a projected future together in which they will continue to rehearse this melody is a harbinger of her all too imminent departure, and her claim to always remember the melody foreshadows the very struggle she will have to remember once in the underworld, and the repetition of learning and relearning that will take place there.

In this opening scene Orpheus and Eurydice are in love and at the beach. Eurydice directs Orpheus to "walk over there" and then tells him, "don't look at me"; the stage directions note that he then "turns his face away from hers and walks" until she says "now—stop," which, according to the stage direction, he does. She runs and jumps in his arms. He doesn't quite catch her and they fall down together" (Ruhl 2006, 334). This scene is repeated but made anew when Orpheus is directed by the lord of the underworld to turn around and walk without looking at Eurydice, until she speaks and he turns to see her. In that scene, as they part ways definitively with her returning to the underworld as he leaves it, they again rehearse their melody, and again, she is unable to produce the rhythm. Orpheus says to Eurydice "remember—I tried to teach you your sense of rhythm—it was—off" (Ruhl 2006, 397). Orpheus wants to linger in memories: "we've known each other for centuries! I want to reminisce" (Ruhl 2006, 399).

As Eurydice is drawn back to the underworld, she recalls "our house … we had two cats/ and two dogs/ and two fish/ that died" (399). In recalling the past, Eurydice recalls the familiar parts of her prior home, while moving toward her unfamiliar, uncanny home. The early scene in which Orpheus and Eurydice fall down together is, as with the uncanny, repeated as familiar yet different. The second time they do not fall together. Eurydice falls to the underworld alone. Departure and return repeat. Eurydice nearly returns from the dead, only to depart again. But this return from the dead is a departure from her father in the underworld, to whom her return is then repeated. Each time the unfamiliarity of death and loss becomes slightly more familiar, the uncanny rendered more homely. For Eurydice, there is no way back to the overworld, but the play presents a clear way ahead, in her rebuilding of herself, her memories, transposing aspects of the familiar to this new location, and re-teaching her father language and their shared memories.

Part of the inherent repetition of theater is that it is performed and re-performed for a new audience every night, and the audience's role is crucial to constituting theater as such: a play is repeated for the audience and the audience receives it, and plays along, in the language game of theater. Much like in Wittgenstein, the individual is part of a community of rule followers in a language game; in theater the individual spectator is a member of an audience, and the theater creates a language game in which actors and audience are a community of rule-followers. This community is engaging not only with the language of theater, but with its space, and importantly, bodily gesture, through the embodied nature of performance, and the embodied nature of being a theatrical audience physically present to witness the performance. Wittgenstein uses theater as a metaphor in his observation that "[o]ne says, for example, to someone who has to play a part on stage. 'Here you must imagine that this man is in pain and is concealing this'—and now we give him no directions, don't tell him what he is *actually* to do. For this reason, too, the suggested analysis is not the point.—We now watch the actor, who is imagining this situation" (Wittgenstein 2009, §393).

Wittgenstein explores the role of gesture in conveying meaning, describing a hypothetical scenario in which "I turn to stone, and my pain goes on…," wondering how to explain the meaning of "pain" to someone who is not sure if they have also experienced it, or if what they each have experienced as "pain" are in fact the same (or similar) experiences. (Wittgenstein 2009, §288). He goes on to say "we'd explain it to him. … Perhaps by means of gestures, or by pricking him with a pin and saying 'See, that's pain!' This explanation of a word, like any other, he might understand rightly, wrongly or not at all. And he will show which by his use of the word, in this as in other cases" (Wittgenstein 2009, §288). In *Eurydice* the title character must continually explain herself to the personified stones, who are like Wittgenstein's subject who has turned to stone. These theatrical stones do not understand the language that Eurydice brings with her to the underworld: she must repeatedly explain to them her meanings, through gesture, performance, and use. Being stones with their own language and language-games, they may understand her "rightly, wrongly or not at all." They may inter-subjectively understand each other "rightly, wrongly, or not at all." As we see throughout the play, Eurydice and the Stones appear to the audience as speaking the same language, but there are recurring instances of their language not matching the other's understanding.

As the audience, we regard these moments of gestural understanding and misunderstanding from the standpoint of a community of knowing viewers. We hold both an omniscient place, knowing (presumably) Eurydice's fate, and understanding the (supposedly different) languages spoken by the Stones, the living, and the dead. Yet we also take on the role of explorer in this particular theatrical world that is opened to us for the first time, unlike the actors for whom the theatrical world has already been repeated in rehearsal or performance many times over. From this position, the audience and actors are engaging with further forms of repetition, rehearsing and performing, watching and re-watching, critically in the company of others.

In her analysis of film, Karen Beckman (2003) underscores the role of watching film critically together, an act that is repeatedly performed within the movie *Whatever Happened to Baby Jane?* in scenes where the characters of the film are watching and re-watching in the company of each other. Beckman suggests the behavior modeled within the movie is illustrative of how film functions: we can watch and re-watch in a community of other viewers. With movies, there is a single fixed version that any audience will see, in perpetuity.[9] Theater affords a different way of re-watching. Instead of one fixed performance that can continually be revisited, theater provides numerous, similar yet distinct performances, which the audience most often will only see once, but which are re-experienced by the actors

[9] Director's cuts and extended version re-releases trouble this point, but they remain fixed instantiations of a product, not entirely plastic ones. That movies shot on film can degrade or even be destroyed further complicates the fixity of any single way of viewing a particular film, but the point holds that film tends to afford a verbatim replica of itself to each viewer.

themselves. While there is an inversion of who the critical re-watchers are between film and theater, what is unique about theater is the possibility of revision: it is repeated, but anew, with the endless potential for rediscovery or seeing differently. Certainly this is limited to not only a particular run of a performance, but the very nature of theater that it is a piece of work that exists in written form and will be revived. Here, the terms of the theater speak to the uncanniness of repetition that a play coming back to the stage is called a "revival"—it is brought back to life.

There are embedded layers of watching in *Eurydice*: the King of the Underworld has a certain omniscient viewership standpoint, yet he is also a subjective, fickle player with his own motivations and desires. The Stones function like an observing Greek chorus. There is an audience watching the action on stage. Theater creates a community of interpreters, in which the audience is brought in to a shared space of watching, and thinking critically, together. Each audience member has his or her own experience with the performance both privately and as part of a community. The community of performed repetition in theater creates the conditions for the repeated opportunity, in the vocabulary of Wittgenstein, for seeing-as differently, and a new dawning of an aspect, with each performance and each viewing.

Conclusion: Staging of Grief

In theatrical repetition, what is important is the act of repeating with the possibility for it to be modified—there is always the opportunity for a new aspect. This may be true within the run of a single play, for an actor to discover a new aspect to reveal in the text or her performance, or this possibility for a new aspect may be part of a play's existence in the world as a piece of theater intended to be repeated, rehearsed, re-imagined, potentially endlessly. There is always the chance for a new dawning of an aspect with a new iteration, staging or dramatic rehearsal. The very fact of re-imagining the myth of Eurydice, as a new play from a new perspective, reveals a dawning of a new aspect. And this is an embodied repetition, in lived experience, phenomenologically, that is unique to theater. The theater not only invites the imagination on the part of those staging a play and those viewing it; its very structure of embodied repetition as the language game of theater itself invites imagination and the engagement with new ways of seeing-as and new dawning of aspects.

Theater also functions according to language-games and repeated tropes of genre including tragedy and comedy. *Eurydice* is an allusion to a classic work of tragedy, yet the play itself is not tragic. It employs comedic elements throughout, existing on the frontier between tragedy and comedy, constantly moving between the two. In reinventing a classic work of tragedy, the play reinvents a response to the skeptical problem Cavell connects to tragedy: that it "is a projection or an enactment of a skeptical problematic" (Cavell 1988, 173), or the problem of acknowledging other minds. *Eurydice* enacts a response by repeatedly inviting and invoking identification between characters and across audience and character, as part of the process of acknowledging losses of both others and the self. Cavell writes about Thoreau's *Walden* being an exercise in "finding ecstasy in the knowledge of loss" (Cavell 1988, 171) and notes that Thoreau wrote in the image of the location of Paradise. *Eurydice* takes us to the underworld, here it is neither heaven nor hell, but the next life—an eternal life—that is the epitome of the nature of uncanny repetition of the ordinary of which Cavell speaks.

In its repetition of the familiar and the uncanny, what is ordinary and eternal in contrast to what is newly seen and seen anew, *Eurydice* reveals, as Wittgenstein would say, what is hidden in plain sight. In this case, what is hidden and uncovered are our own ideas and feelings of grief, loss, and mourning. While the play may help us confront our own mortal selves as mortal subjects, it most importantly demands of us to see how we respond to the loss of another—which inherently contains a part of the loss of the self. At the same it invites our identification with a character who is dead, trying on the experience of being dead in ways only the imagination and fiction can allow us to access (at least while living as embodied beings). We may keep grief hidden, yet it is hidden in plain sight, always around us, in the repeated experiences of the ordinary and the uncanny.

Bibliography

Al-Shamma, James. *Sarah Ruhl: A Critical Study of the Plays*. McFarland, 2011.

Beckman, Karen. *Vanishing Women: Magic, Film, and Feminism*. Duke UP, 2003.

Cavell, Stanley. "Knowing and Acknowledging." *Must We Mean What We Say?* Cambridge UP, 1969, pp. 238–266.

———. "The Uncanniness of the Ordinary." *In Quest of the Ordinary: Lines of Skepticism and Romanticism*. U of Chicago P, 1988.

Freud, Sigmund. *The Uncanny*. Translated by David McLintock. Penguin Books, 2003.

Lanphier, Elizabeth. "Witnessing Illness: Phenomenology of Photographic Self Portraiture." *Bodies and Transitions in the Health Humanities* edited by Lisa DeTora and Stephanie Hilger. Routledge Press, 2020, pp. 132–142.

Moran, Richard. "The Expression of Feeling in Imagination." *Philosophical Review*, vol. 103, no. 1, 1994, pp. 75–106.

Ruhl, Sarah. *The Clean House and Other Plays (Eurydice, Late: A Cowboy Song, Melancholy Play)*. Theater Communications Group, 2006.

Wittgenstein, Ludwig. *Last Writings on the Philosophy of Psychology*. Vol. 1. Edited by G.H. von Wright and Heikki Nyman, translated by C.G Luckhardt and Maximillian A.E. AUE. U of Chicago P, 1982.

———. *Philosophical Investigations*. Revised Fourth Edition. Translated by G.E.M. Anscombe, P.M.S. Hacker and Joachim Schulte. Edited by P.M.S Hacker and Joachim Schulte. Wiley-Blackwell, 2009.

PART II

Envisioning the Other

"Why Should I Imagine Such a Thing?": Suffering in Michael Haneke's *Amour*

Derek Ettensohn

Introduction

Georges and Anne Laurent (Louis Trintignant and Emmanuelle Riva), the two elderly protagonists of Michael Haneke's *Amour* (2012), arrive home from a concert to discover that someone has attempted to break into their apartment with a screwdriver. Anne asks Georges, "Imagine if we were here, in our beds, and someone broke in." To which Georges replies, "Why should I imagine such a thing?" (*Amour* 06:10). While Georges poses this question in response to Anne's comment, his question frames a film that invites viewers to witness the pain and suffering that results from Anne's subsequent illness. Though the question could be read as an effort to downplay Anne's fears or to conceal Georges's own, it suggests the limited value in imagining such an event. Certainly, whatever he or Anne can imagine could never equal the fear, panic, and sense of vulnerability should they find an actual intruder in their house. Read through Georges's

D. Ettensohn (✉)
Sewanee: The University of the South, Sewanee, TN, USA
e-mail: dmettens@sewanee.edu

J. Cressman et al. (eds.), *Envisioning Embodiment in the Health Humanities*, Sustainable Development Goals Series,
https://doi.org/10.1007/978-3-031-49807-7_8

response, *Amour* also asks why an audience should view the tremendous suffering on screen as Anne falls ill. This essay uses an analysis of *Amour* to consider how and why we read, view, and imagine stories of suffering and then to reflect on how these activities can be framed in the health humanities classroom.

Amour is a difficult film to watch. Considering the suffering on screen, why, to revise Georges's question, should we view such a thing? The film seems to invite such questioning. For example, in an article for *The New York Review of Books*, "A Masterpiece You Might Not Want to See," Francis Prose writes:

> *Amour* is a love story all right, or at least the final chapter of one. In its intensity, its unflinching determination to track what happens to the dying and those around them, it recalls "The Death of Ivan Ilyich." But while I have read Tolstoy's story several times and expect to read it again, I can't imagine wanting to see *Amour* a second time. Why would I voluntarily put myself through the awfulness of watching the scenes in which the couple struggles to navigate the suddenly staggering demands of the wheelchair, the knife and fork, the toilet? (Prose)

In his review of the film, Roger Ebert similarly asks, "Why would we want to see such a film, however brilliantly it has been made?" (Ebert). These reactions were largely shared by the students in my seminar "Health, Illness, and the Humanities." While students found it an important and moving work, none of them would recommend the film to a friend, let alone to their parents, relatives, or grandparents who might be experiencing prolonged illness firsthand. Prose concludes her piece on *Amour* with a similar sentiment: "The experience (and the courage required) is impressive, but the view is so unrelentingly brutal that we may well wonder why we are seeing it sooner than we have to" (Prose). In realistically portraying Anne's decline and death, *Amour* appears "brutal" precisely because, like the actual experience of illness, it offers little guidance to make meaning out of Anne's suffering.

The "unrelentingly brutal" portrayal of Anne's illness begins with the stroke she suffers the morning after the attempted burglary; the film captures her pride, despondency, shame, suffering, and her death. We learn of Anne's diagnosis when her daughter Eva (Isabelle Huppert) visits Georges at the apartment: Anne's carotid artery is blocked and, after an unsuccessful operation, there is a strong possibility of another debilitating stroke.

Despite this diagnosis, Anne and Georges attempt to maintain their independence. Anne's refusal to return to the hospital thrusts Georges into the role of a caregiver who must determine how to respond to Anne's suffering. Anne, despite returning from the hospital unable to walk or use her right hand, initially tries to maintain some semblance of her former self; she tells her husband not to fuss over her: "I'm not a cripple. You can easily leave me alone for a minute" (*Amour* 26:50). While these early scenes capture the couple's determined and proud independence, the reality of Anne's illness and their dependence on others provokes a growing despondency, particularly for Anne. Though much of the film focuses on the ethical concerns confronting Georges as he responds to his wife's suffering, Anne announces her own distress at how her illness affects the couple: "There's no reason to go on living. I know it can only get worse. Why must I inflict that on us? On you and me" (*Amour* 42:45). Though we witness some improvement in Anne and happier exchanges, the audience, like Anne, knows that another stroke remains likely. Its arrival and Anne's subsequent decline is nevertheless a shock that forces Georges and the viewer to confront Anne's suffering as she struggles to speak or eat and becomes bedridden. As viewers we are in the position of voyeurs, watching Anne's discomfort as nurses arrive to take her to the bathroom, give her a shower, or help her with food. In many of these scenes, Anne can only articulate the word *mal*, crying out repeatedly. We witness Anne's pain and Georges's growing distress at her suffering until, near the end of the film, Georges smothers Anne. Presented through a long take from a stationary camera, this surprising act of violence is also framed as an act of love and mercy.

With so much suffering on screen, the film and its characters question whether or not Anne's anguishing condition should be shown. Late in the film, Georges initially refuses to allow Eva to see her mother. In justifying his refusal, Georges recounts the daily routine necessary to manage Anne's suffering, telling Eva that "none of all that deserves to be shown" (*Amour* 1:37:35). Yet, the film invades the private spaces that Georges would like closed off from even his daughter. In doing so, *Amour* raises critical and ethical questions about how art represents pain, suffering, and death as well as the value that we attribute to such representations. I open the essay by highlighting the important representation of illness, suffering, and care in *Amour*, before arguing that Haneke's refusal to ascribe meaning to illness and suffering refocuses our attention on the questions of narrative and imagination that have been central to narrative ethics, narrative medicine, and the health humanities more broadly. When read through Georges's skepticism toward the imagination, *Amour*, I argue, stresses both the limits of the imagination and the value of storytelling in moving its characters to action. I conclude by reflecting on the position of *Amour* in the health humanities classroom as students reflect on their own expectations for art, literature, and cinema, articulating how and to what end they believe illness, pain, and suffering should be represented.

Illness, Suffering, and Care in *Amour*

Critics have sought to answer the question of why we should view the suffering and pain in *Amour* through a variety of disciplinary angles. These include responses from film scholars like Melanie Robson who show how the formal elements of *Amour*, particularly Haneke's long takes, pull the viewer into the central moral dilemma of the film. Approaching the film through Jean-Luc Nancy's philosophy, Milosz Paul Rosinski emphasizes the political and ethical concerns around death in the film, while Taylor Worley grounds his analysis in theology to argue that the film arrives at a "theology of death" that reveals "love—self-giving, self-risking, self-shattering love—alone can lead us through death" (Worley 19). Of particular concern in these accounts is the ethics of Georges's final act, read either as an act of mercy or as an act of selfishness.[1] While the startling scene where Georges smothers Anne remains central to any interpretation of *Amour*, the question of how we read Georges's actions must be situated in how the film transmits the experience of illness, suffering, and caregiving. The film seems to confound an effort to make meaning out of Anne's pain or to displace that pain and suffering onto structural factors, something Haneke has noted in interviews:

> I wanted to avoid making my film a "social drama." There have been enough films that present these themes as a social drama, that deal with context and environment, with hospitals, ambulances, and doctors. That's not what I

[1] Roy Grundmann notes that the ethical dilemma in the film is not between choosing life and death, but how "such a choice, even when fueled by radical compassion and even in the arena of romantic love is never completely altruistic" (Grundmann par. 2). Grundmann's suggestion that Georges's act can be read as "selfishness incarnate" situates the film within Haneke's body of work, particularly his representation of violence (par. 2). This contrasts with critics such as Moira Weigel who view the film as break from Haneke's approach to violence (Weigel par. 24).

> was trying to do. I didn't want to make a social drama, but an existential drama that deals with the question: "How do I cope with the suffering of a loved one?" (Qtd. in Worley 2)

Largely remaining within the confines of the couple's apartment, *Amour* captures not only the claustrophobic reduction of the world through illness, but also the private confrontation of illness and suffering that occurs at an existential level.

As Haneke's comment suggests, the film largely centers on Georges's experience of Anne's illness and his efforts to come to terms with her suffering. While the audience witnesses Anne's suffering, it is not asked to imagine this suffering directly. In fact, as I will argue later, the film seems to suggest the limits of such imagination in favor of a recognition of her experience through storytelling. Rather, the audience is placed in the position of Georges, who struggles with how he should respond to his wife's pain. Even before the later stroke takes away Anne's ability to speak clearly, Georges finds himself at a loss for how to respond to his wife's experience. Immediately after returning to their apartment Anne asks Georges to promise her that he will never take her back to the hospital. Georges hesitantly responds, "What can I say?," promising nothing as Anne interrupts to prevent him from explaining further (*Amour* 25:45). One can sense Georges's anguish as he must comfort his wife and confront the possibility that she will need to return to the hospital for care.

Torn between his desire to comply with his wife's wishes and his own sense of obligation to provide her care, Georges's difficulty in coping with Anne's suffering only grows following the stroke that leaves her bedridden and unable to easily communicate. Georges witnesses the indignities that Anne is made to suffer and the challenge she has in expressing her will—her repeated screams of "*mal*," for example, or her refusal to eat or drink. Though the nurse dismisses Anne's cries as meaningless, her assurances are of little comfort as Georges and the audience must determine whether this explanation willfully ignores Anne's labored effort to communicate. Anne's refusal to drink offers Georges no such ambiguity as she rejects his efforts at care. When Georges loses his temper with Anne and slaps her in the face after her refusal, he forces a confrontation between Anne's will for death and his own obligations to care.

In its representation of Georges's effort to cope with his wife's suffering, Haneke's film memorably captures how illness violates the space of the home, transforms daily routines, and alienates its characters from their sense of self.[2] Following the opening credits, the film begins with an explosive noise as police and firemen break down the doors of Georges and Anne's apartment. Entering the apartment, they find the corpse of Anne on a bed strewn with flowers. Though Anne imagines a thief breaking into her home, it is instead illness that violates the most intimate spaces of her home, particularly the bedroom. Shortly before Anne returns home from her failed operation we see two men arrive to install a new mattress, beginning the transformation of the couple's bedroom. As her illness advances Anne's bedside table accumulates the objects necessary for her daily care: tissues, latex gloves, a bedpan, lotions, buckets, a carton of incontinence pads, etc. The relative clutter of the bedroom during Anne's illness contrasts with the ordered bedroom of the opening scene of the film as, following her death, Georges has removed all the markers of Anne's illness. Though Anne's death is the climax of *Amour*, the film continues for nearly an additional fifteen minutes, following Georges as he attempts to recover the home by banishing the signs of illness. At the end of the film, he drifts into memories of his late wife before sealing up the apartment and walking out of the film to an unknown fate.[3]

Through its focus on Georges's competing obligations to his wife and the sense of violation and loss of self that it captures through illness as home invasion, *Amour* offers a valuable representation of illness and suffering. Despite this moving representation, *Amour* confounds an audience's expectations for making meaning out of the experience of suffering it portrays. As Prose notes of the film's grim portrayal of Anne's decline, "there's no transcendence in *Amour*, no comfort" (Prose). Similarly, Moira Weigel characterizes the film as a "passion play that holds out no religious consolation" (Weigel par. 6). In denying transcendence or consolation, Haneke's film suggests an ethical position that recognizes the limits of our understanding of suffering. The film, Robson observes, further plays with proximity to demonstrate how being too close or too distanced from Anne and Georges's situation affects how characters and, in turn, viewers interpret the couple's dilemma (Robson 109). *Amour* relies

[2] For more on the domestic space in Haneke's work see David Sorfa's "Uneasy Domesticity in the Films of Michael Haneke" (2006) and Catherine Wheatley's "Domestic Invasion: Michael Haneke and Home Audiences" (2011).

[3] While we don't know the fate of Georges by the end of *Amour*, Trintignant plays another version of Georges Laurent in Haneke's 2017 film *Happy End*. Trintignant's elderly character repeatedly tries to end his life in the later film and tells his granddaughter the story of how he smothered his late wife to relieve her suffering.

on a similar aesthetic as Haneke's other films—long takes with a static camera—that forces the audience to generate meaning. Detailing how Haneke's films places "the burden of ethical reflection on the viewer," Oliver Speck notes that "the viewer is responsibilized by the film to perform shifts of frame of reference him or herself" (Speck 10). The film refuses to guide its audience toward an interpretation or argument, rather forcing them to rely on and interrogate their own frames of reference. Haneke's refusal to guide a viewer toward meaning, along with the frequent questioning within the film of what should be shown or imagined, draw the viewer into a consideration of how one can ethically construct meaning out of another's experience of illness and suffering.

Imagination and Storytelling in *Amour*

In inviting us to view such suffering and pain while withholding an interpretive framework to understand it, *Amour* suggests the difficulty in deriving a meaning or narrative from the experience of illness. While many texts within the canon of the health humanities construct a narrative of illness, Haneke's film places that work onto the viewer as they seek to understand Anne's pain and Georges's final act. This makes the film particularly useful in pushing students to consider the imaginative and ethical work demanded of narrative medicine in its confrontation with illness and suffering. Central to the work of narrative medicine is the role of the imagination. In delineating the relation of narrative ethics as a precursor to narrative medicine, Arthur Frank argues that narrative ethics focuses on a pedagogy that helps "people become capable of new imaginations of themselves and, crucially, of others and their imagination of what they must do" (Frank S16). Further stressing the importance of the imagination, Frank continues, "the narrative ethicist imagines life as multiple points of view, each reflecting a distinct imagination and each more or less capable of comprehending other points of view and how they imagine" (S16). Haneke's film productively evaluates the work of the imagination central to accounts, such as Frank's, of narrative ethics and narrative medicine. Throughout *Amour*, Haneke suggests a generative limit to our feeling with another or our imagination of another's experience. The film, however, reveals the limits of the imagination only to establish the value of storytelling in orienting Georges toward ethical action.

Amour offers an important representation of the experience of illness, aging, and care-taking, though, perhaps most critically, its refusal to indicate how we should generate meaning from its representation of suffering refocuses our attention on the role of imagination and storytelling to produce ethical action. While early in the film Georges dismisses imagining "such a thing" as a burglar entering their apartment, *Amour* invites and then contests the value of imagining Anne's suffering and Georges's increasingly frustrated care. When Anne tells Georges that she wishes to die after he finds her huddled on the ground near an open window, Georges replies, "Put yourself in my shoes. Haven't you ever thought it could happen to me, too?" (*Amour* 43:15). Invoking the language of empathy, Georges asks Anne to imagine his own position as a caretaker. Anne responds, "Of course I have. But imagination and reality have little in common" (43:20). Anne, the character who earlier asked her husband to imagine the horror of a break in, now observes the gap between imagination and reality. Instead, it is Georges who asks Anne to put herself in his place. Anne's response suggests that she has imagined their roles reversing, though ultimately that imagination has little relation to her current reality, much like his imagination of her condition cannot capture her own reality.

Amour appears to create an impasse as the audience is invited to witness Anne's suffering and imagine the predicaments that Georges faces in providing her care, while the film's characters stress the limits of such imagining. The film, however, does not resign itself to the incommensurability of Anne and Georges's experiences. Rather, it stresses a form of imagining that clarifies the imaginative work of Frank's narrative ethics or the practice of narrative medicine, which Rita Charon has advocated for as "medicine practiced with these narrative skills of recognizing, absorbing, interpreting, and being moved by the stories of illness" (Charon 4). Charon notes that "narrative knowledge" allows a person to understand "the plight of another by participating in his or her story with complex skills of imagination, interpretation, and recognition. With such knowledge, we enter others' narrative worlds and accept them—at least provisionally—as true" (Charon 9–10). Charon highlights the importance of the work of imagination and narrative in an anecdote about a patient named Luz who had asked Charon to sign a disability form due to headaches. Initially irritated at the request, Charon is later upset about how she handled the incident and writes a story about the encounter. Without all the facts about Luz, Charon creates a background story for Luz that involves her moving to Manhattan to pursue a career in modeling. While she imagines Luz to have a story that captures Luz's desire to leave home, the reality that Charon later uncovers—an abusive father—is far more urgent. Though Charon does not spend much time reflecting on why she had imagined Luz as a model, her narrative appears to be framed through common stories of youthful ambition in the big city. Charon turns to an almost clichéd tale, though one that nevertheless opens her to Luz's actual story. What is remarkable about Charon's anecdote is not how well she is able to imagine Luz's story, but rather how even in revealing the limits of her imagination the very act of creating a narrative—however inaccurate—leads Charon to action.

While *Amour* appears quite removed from Charon's concerns with narrative medicine and clinical practice, Haneke's film stresses the challenges of interpreting illness and the role of storytelling in generating ethical action. In both Charon and Frank's models, imagining leads to dialogue between physician and patient as well as between the patient and others. However, in Haneke's film the focus remains on the relationship between an elderly couple to reveal the consequential struggle to understand the meaning of the suffering of those with whom we are most intimate. The film begins with the invitation to imagine, yet such imaginings lead to a failure of dialogue as we witness several abortive attempts to discuss Anne's condition and to collectively reimagine the couple's future. Yet, the film remains invested in stories, though it questions how we hear these stories, particularly of those who cannot fully communicate their suffering. While we are invited to witness Anne's suffering, we are warned about the limits of how we might imagine both her suffering and the toll of care-taking on Georges. Nevertheless, "imagining such a thing"—however distant from the reality of that thing—will, as Charon suggests of storytelling, be a tool for locating the truth (Charon 6). In *The Wounded Storyteller* Frank describes narrative ethics as building an empathy that is not "internalizing the feelings of the other," but, citing Jodi Halpern, is in "'resonance' with the other" (158). In this mode of empathetic imagining, Frank notes that "the other's self-story does not become my own, but I develop sufficient resonance with that story so that I can feel its nuances and anticipate changes in plot" (158). In Haneke's film, storytelling helps move Georges to perform the difficult work of distinguishing his and Anne's experience of her illness, guiding him away from the shared story of their life together and toward a better understanding of her condition and her desires that ultimately leads to action.

Georges relates the most consequential story in *Amour* to Anne right before he ends her life. Anne's cries bring Georges to their bedroom and, when he cannot comfort her or locate the source of her pain, he turns to a story of his time at camp when he was ten years old. Recounting the daily program of the camp, the terrible food he refused to eat, and the punishment he received as a result, Georges shares a story of private suffering that he can only communicate with his mother through code: “I had to write her every week. I had to send her a postcard. If I was enjoying camp, I had to draw flowers on it. If not, stars. She kept that card. It was covered in stars” (*Amour* 1:47:15–1:47:40). Following his punishment for refusing to eat, George falls ill with diphtheria and is placed in an isolation ward. When his mother does come to visit, Georges tells Anne, she “could only wave at me through a window.” It is unclear how we should interpret this story, or if analyzing it risks diverting our focus from Georges's subsequent actions. The story emphasizes Georges's resistance to a regime of bodily discipline at the camp, his difficulty in articulating his displeasure, and his ultimate isolation and separation from his mother due to illness. Melanie Robson suggests that Georges's “story of miscommunication is designed to sympathise with wife's inability to communicate” (Robson 104). While I agree that Georges's narration forms an identification with Anne, I would argue that it is not an identification with Anne's difficulty to communicate, but rather a belated recognition of what she has been communicating. Georges's story seems to create a dual identification as he recalls the housemaster who punished him for refusing to eat and his own anger at the efforts of the camp to keep the campers busy, training their bodies to “nip in the bud any possible pubescent impulses” (*Amour* 1:46:15). Narrating the efforts of the housemaster to control the body and orient it toward healthy productivity and his own resistance to this routine, Georges makes visible Anne's similar resistance. The story allows him to reimagine his role and to separate Anne's illness and suffering from his own experience of her illness. Furthermore, the story relates an effort to communicate that does not attempt to fully represent or transmit an experience. The stars that the young Georges draws relate only displeasure and suffering, foregoing the specifics of the experience that, at that point, cannot be transmitted. His mother does not know the details of what is going on at the camp, yet she acts on their message. Anne's repetition of *mal*, like the stars, cannot fully transmit her pain and suffering, yet her cries invite an imagining of her suffering. Georges may not be able to imagine the specifics of Anne's pain, yet he too acts.

Haneke in the Health Humanities Classroom

Haneke's film stresses the work of storytelling and imagination that leads Georges to move beyond feeling to action. In the health humanities classroom, *Amour* powerfully represents aging, illness, suffering, and caregiving while further chronicling Georges's difficult movement from imagining to acting at the end of the film. Georges's decision to act aligns with Haneke's concern, voiced in interviews, that "[w]hat we do for another person is more important than what we feel for them" ("Michael Haneke on *Amour*"). Though there remain questions about the ethics of Georges's actions, the film offers its audience a model of imagining and narrating that arrives at new insights even if it does not arrive at an understanding of the experience of Anne's suffering. While operating in a different frame, this complements Charon's sense that what she imagines about Luz is not the truth, but rather a "hypothesis...with which to get to the truth" (Charon 6). Moving away from the relationship between medical professional and patient, Haneke's film provides insight into the difficulty of imagining new narratives when coping with the suffering of a loved one. The audience witnesses Georges's struggles, while it too is asked to interpret and frame the suffering that it sees on screen. Though we might not get to an ultimate truth about Georges and Anne while watching *Amour*, Haneke, in inviting us to "imagine such a thing," gets us closer to truths about love, death, illness, suffering, and care—truths that are all framed through narratives. This is the final move that I see the film making and one that tries to answer the question that Georges poses at the beginning of the film.

Haneke's film emphasizes how the stories we have heard and the images we have seen mediate how we view ourselves and imagine others. This begins with the casting of Riva and Trintignant, two legendary French actors that pull us out of the imagined world of the film through its intertextual affiliations. It extends, of course, to the examples of storytelling in the film and the recognition that these stories are often misremembered and incomplete. While stressing the limits of the imagination, *Amour* asks us to imagine bodily pain, suffering, and death within the context of our daily lives. It does so, however, with the knowledge that the specifics of what we have seen will likely be forgotten, though the sensation the film has produced, and our retelling of these sensations, will continue to inform how we confront illness and the end of life.

Early in the film, shortly after returning home from the hospital, Georges tells Anne about a trip to the cinema when he was a boy. Though he fails to recall the film's plot—a sentimental romance—he tells Anne that "I remember being overcome with emotion when I came out of the film. It took me a while to calm down" (*Amour* 32:45). What seems to imprint this moment in Georges's memory, however, is the retelling of the film to a young man who lived in his grandmother's building: "I started telling him the story, and, as I did so, the emotion bubbled up again. I wasn't going to cry in front of him, but I couldn't help myself. I stood there in tears in the courtyard, telling him the whole damn story" (33:15–34:05). When Anne asks about the young man's reaction, Georges simply states that he cannot remember. What he does recall is his various emotions, his sense of shame for crying during both the film and his retelling of it. All that remains of the film, Georges suggests, is sentiment, emotion, and the call to imagine that story as, in some way, his own. All the while, new stories are introduced through the retelling. It is not the initial viewing that Georges focuses on, but rather its retelling and the frame that he has put on that retelling. *Amour*, as Lynn Higgins observes, is concerned with memory, though it emphasizes "less the memory's cognitive context than the event's subjective and affective afterlife, even its sensory perseveration" (Higgins 87). While Higgins's essay centers around sound, *Amour* more broadly suggests the importance of storytelling, the affect it creates, and the frames that we place around stories as we reinterpret them within the context of our own lives.

The value of *Amour* for the health humanities class emerges not only through its presentation of Anne's illness and death or Georges's use of storytelling to arrive at action, but also through its consideration of the frames that shape imagination and narrative. Much as the film emphasizes the frames that we place on experience as well as how stories shape these frames, teaching *Amour* highlights the framing work performed by the texts that surround it in the classroom. In my humanities seminar, *Amour* followed two texts frequently taught in the health humanities: Leo Tolstoy's *The Death of Ivan Ilyich* and Margaret Edson's *Wit*. Through the insights gained by the suffering protagonists of Tolstoy's Ivan Ilyich and Edson's Vivian Bearing, these texts offer didactic narratives of illness and suffering that Haneke's film studiously avoids. Rather than guiding a viewer through how to make meaning out of pain and suffering, as Edson's play so notably does, Haneke insists that the viewer takes responsibility over both locating meaning and then evaluating how they arrived at this meaning. What remains from Haneke's film is not the comforting movement toward transcendence, as seen in *Wit* or *The Death of Ivan Ilyich*, but rather the sensation of claustrophobia, discomfort, and horror. Perhaps this is why, as Prose notes, Tolstoy's work invites repeated readings, while Haneke's does not—the discomfiting feeling *Amour* creates remains long after viewing it.

Placed into dialogue with Tolstoy and Edson, *Amour* generates conversations about the aims of art and literature and the responsibility of the artist in making meaning out of human experience. Haneke's film openly questions why we should imagine illness, suffering, and death before we must experience them in our own lives. While the film may not invite rewatching, the sensations it creates stays in the memory and invites reimagining and reframing. In the health humanities classroom, I have argued, the film can productively engage with work on narrative ethics and the related field of narrative medicine as it represents the difficulty of locating a narrative and meaning in illness and suffering. The film, moreover, opens up the space to discuss the role of storytelling, imagination, and ethical action that fosters a deeper understanding of the challenges of attending to the suffering of another person. Finally, *Amour* leaves open multiple readings that productively reveal our own attitudes toward illness, suffering, and death, raising important questions regarding why and how they should be represented.

Bibliography

Charon, Rita. *Narrative Medicine*. Oxford UP, 2006.

Ebert, Roger. Review of *Amour*, by Michael Haneke. *RogerEbert.com*, 9 Jan. 2013, https://www.rogerebert.com/reviews/amour-2013. Web. 8 Nov. 2022.

Frank, Arthur W. "Narrative Ethics as Dialogical Story-Telling." *Narrative Ethics: The Role of Stories in Bioethics*, a special report, *Hastings Center Report*, vol. 44, no. 1, Jan.–Feb. 2014, pp. S16–S20.

———. *The Wounded Storyteller*. 2nd ed., The U of Chicago P, 2013.

Grundmann, Roy. "Love, Death, Truth—*Amour*." *Senses of Cinema*, Dec. 2012, http://sensesofcinema.com/2012/feature-articles/love-death-truth-amour/. Web. 8 Nov. 2022.

Haneke, Michael, director. *Amour*. Sony Pictures Classic, 2012.

———. *Happy End*. Sony Pictures Classics, 2017.

———. "Michael Haneke on Amour." Interview by Dave Calhoun. *Time Out Dubai*, 4 Dec. 2012, https://www.timeoutdubai.com/movies/movies-features/37227-michael-haneke-on-amour. Web. 8 Nov. 2022.

Higgins, Lynn. "Becoming a Song: Sound, Memory, and Cinema History in Michael Haneke's *Amour*." *South Central Review*, vol. 33, no. 2, Summer 2016, pp. 80–95.
Prose, Francine. "A Masterpiece You Might Not Want to See." *The New York Review of Books*, 7 Jan. 2013, https://www.nybooks.com/daily/2013/01/07/haneke-film-not-to-see/. Web. 8 Nov. 2022.
Robson, Melanie. "Complicity, Intimacy, and Distance: Re-examining the Active Viewer in Michael Haneke's *Amour*." *Studies in European Cinema*, vol. 14, no. 2, 2017, pp. 103–117.
Rosinksi, Milosz Paul. "Touching Nancy's Ethics: Death in Michael Haneke's *Amour*." *Studies in French Cinema*, vol. 15, no. 2, April 2015, pp. 180–196.
Sorfa, David. "Uneasy domesticity in the films of Michael Haneke." *Studies in European Cinema*, vol. 3, no. 2, 2006, pp. 93–104.
Speck, Oliver C. *Funny Frames: The Filmic Concepts of Michael Haneke*. Continuum International Publishing Group, 2010.
Weigel, Moira. "Sadomodernism: Haneke in Furs." *n +1*, issue 16: Double Bind, Spring 2013, http://nplusonemag.com/sadomodernism/. Web. 8 Nov. 2022.
Wheatley, Catherine. "Domestic Invasion: Michael Haneke and Home Audiences." *The Cinema of Michael Haneke: Europe Utopia*. Edited by Ben McCann and David Sorfa, Wallflower Press, 2011, pp. 10–23.
Worley, Taylor. "Losing Touch: A Theology of Death for Michael Haneke's *Amour*." *Religions*, vol. 7, no. 12, 30 Nov. 2016, pp. 1–20.

The Myth of France: Identity Construction Through Migration in Young Adult Francophone Literature

Kaitlyn Waller

In the beginning of Gisèle Pineau's *Un Papillon dans la Cité* (1992), ten-year-old protagonist Félicie must leave her native Guadeloupe to join her mother in France. Flying across the Atlantic for the first time, she anxiously wonders what to expect when she lands in the outskirts of Paris. Seventeen years later, Insa Sané simultaneously recreates and distorts a similar scene as Djiraël, the cynical, occasionally crass, teen protagonist of *Sarcelles-Dakar* (2009), makes the opposite journey, flying overseas from the Parisian banlieues to Senegal for his father's funeral. Djiraël hasn't returned to his home country since he was a small child, but feels confident that not much has changed—including himself.

In some ways, *Sarcelles–Dakar* is a reversal of *Un Papillon dans la Cité*. Rather than trying to adapt to a new country like Félicie, Djiraël is trying to reconnect with his native one. While Félicie wants to reconnect with her mother, who left her when she was a baby, Djiraël wants to find closure

K. Waller (✉)
Independent Scholar, Seogwipo, South Korea

J. Cressman et al. (eds.), *Envisioning Embodiment in the Health Humanities*, Sustainable Development Goals Series,
https://doi.org/10.1007/978-3-031-49807-7_9

with the father who stayed behind while Djiraël moved away. Yet these young adult novels also have fundamental similarities: both feature protagonists whose coming-of-age stories are set against the complexities of migration, specifically via France. Furthermore, in both novels, France—or the myth of France—influences and fragments their development of identity and belonging.

The basic coming-of-age story is a classic tradition in young adult literature, a genre already preoccupied with the search for identity and belonging. Indeed, in his analysis of the genre, Aidan Chambers concludes that young adult literature "must inevitably deal with maturation, de-identification, and with questions of identity and life-purpose, because these are endemic in youthness" (281). When examining young adult novels through the lens of migration narratives, these questions of identity become even more pronounced. Elia Michelle Lafuente writes that "literature dealing with migrancy emphasizes the migrant's unsettled identity in relationship to both sites" (43). Just as the young adult navigates independence from the family, so too does the migrant navigate distance from his or her home culture. In young adult narratives of migration, then, this displacement collides and compounds in the adolescent protagonist, who becomes "other" from their changing bodies, familial structures, and home cultures. The young adult migrant must simultaneously forge a new, hybridized cultural identity *and* develop their identity as an independent adult. In the case of Francophone literature, the location of France adds yet another fascinating dimension, as the country itself undergoes the same identity deconstruction and transformation as the protagonists.

In *Un Papillon dans la Cité* and *Sarcelles-Dakar*, the depiction of France is not constant. Indeed, France becomes a site riddled with seemingly irreconcilable partialities, not fully knowable by either the migrant protagonists who make it their home or their extended families; furthermore, viewing France through the lens of the young adult migrant serves to detach readers from their own potentially idealistic conceptions of the country. This multifaceted and conflicting identity is not new to literature; post-colonial criticism frequently dissects France's complicated relationship to its former and current citizens and subjects. Frantz Fanon, for example, scathingly observed the mirage of French superiority among his contemporaries: "Le Noir qui connaît la métropole est un demi-dieu … Beaucoup d'Antillais, après un séjour plus ou moins long dans la métropole, reviennent se faire consacrer" (15).[1] More recently, Omar Ba, in *Je suis venu, j'ai vu, je n'y crois plus*, urges young Africans to reconsider the myth of the European El Dorado (Lesne, 206). Significantly, young adult literature also captures the complexity of the myth of France, often elegantly broaching the same themes driving postcolonial theorists.

As the respective protagonists of Pineau's *Un Papillon dans la Cité* and Sané's *Sarcelles-Dakar* undergo their own coming-of-age stories, traveling between France and their home countries, Félicie and Djiraël may initially see France through a narrow lens. This viewpoint serves as a foundation in their own nascent development; both feel like they embody a distinctly *other* identity (primarily as Guadeloupian and Senegalese) that is incapable of fully connecting with a French one. With time, however, this becomes muddled. Their growing awareness of the intricacies of the world allow them to more easily embrace the subtleties and contradictions of modern geopolitical realities, transnational identities, and globally connected diasporas.

Félicie's and Djiraël's stories are thus focused on movement, as the two learn to constantly navigate the hybridization of multiple cultures, and find contentment and meaning in liminal spaces and otherness. The present chapter will discuss this transformative process through three primary lenses. First, I will present an analysis of the protagonists' coming-of-age, and how the context of migration destabilizes and transforms the conception of a simple, linear journey to self-discovery and adulthood. Second, I will examine how matrilineal or parental connections influence both conceptions and constructions of identity. Finally, I focus on how even in these French young adult novels, the protagonists exist in fragmented, multilingual spaces. Throughout each section, the supposed hegemony of France and French is challenged and transfigured as the protagonists grow to understand themselves and their places in a larger diaspora. While France—or the shifting myth of France—is inextricable from Félicie and Djiraël's identities, it does not ultimately dominate them. Rather, the protagonists must learn to simultaneously re-imagine the self as an embodiment of impermanent cultural, geopolitical, and personal identity *and* extend this conceptualization to the other—recognizing that no one identity is so simple as to be fully understood by another.

[1] "The black man who knows mainland France is a demigod ... Many of them, after a stay in metropolitan France, come home to be deified."

Un Papillon dans la Cité and *Sarcelles-Dakar*

Before analyzing the novels further, it is necessary to briefly outline the general plot of each. While *Un Papillon dans la Cité* was published and set in 1992, it feels as contemporary as *Sarcelles-Dakar*, published in 2009. Both novels fall into the young adult genre as defined by Chambers, and feature Francophone countries juxtaposed with mainland France. Crucially, each novel also highlights a character leaving ***and returning*** to their home country, allowing for a nuanced analysis of their growth and development.

Félicie, who is ten years old at the beginning of *Un Papillon dans la Cité*, was born in Guadeloupe; she is thus both a citizen and an outsider to mainland France. In the beginning of the novel, she lives with her grandmother, Man Ya, in an almost Edenic paradise in rural Guadeloupe. Soon, however, she receives a letter from her mother, Aurélie, explaining that Félicie must travel to Paris to live with her family: Aurélie, her stepfather Papa Jo, and her stepbrother Michel. Félicie is a bright and optimistic child; she settles into life in the faubourgs of Paris, rises to the top of her class, and becomes good friends with a boy in her neighborhood named Mohamed. Although she adjusts relatively well to Paris, she still misses Man Ya and Guadeloupe, and dreams of showing Mohamed her home. She struggles even more when, after winter vacation, Mohamed seems to have drifted away from her. However, after Félicie's teacher announces a class trip to Guadeloupe, Félicie is able to rekindle her friendship with Mohamed. In Guadeloupe, she shows him everything she loves about her home: the sea, the foods, and, above all else, Man Ya.

In the novel's final scene, Félicie and Mohamed return to Paris, where they are greeted by her mother, Papa Jo, and Michel. This ending echoes the novel's first pages—Félicie traveling to Paris. The similar setting makes Félicie's growth all the more apparent: by the end of the novel, she is more mature, confident, and secure in her place, both in her family and the world. In some ways, her story follows the traditional trajectory of coming-of-age stories: leaving the safety and security of home, encountering more of the real world, and beginning to transition from childhood to adolescence and, eventually, adulthood. The circularity of the structure, however, also subverts the linearity of her path and suggests that Félicie's ultimate identity will not be unidimensional.

Like *Un Papillon dans la Cité*, *Sarcelles-Dakar* ends where it begins: in the Parisian banlieues. *Sarcelles-Dakar* follows the story of seventeen-year-old Djiraël as he (reluctantly) returns to Senegal for the funeral of his father—his first time back since he immigrated to France when he was five years old, and a chance to "[s]e familiariser à nouveau avec le quartier" (68).[2] His goal of refamiliarization is more complicated than he originally assumes. In many ways, Dakar hasn't changed from his last visit. Djiraël, on the other hand, has. He learns that he is now considered a "francenabé," "un petit Sénégalais de France qui vient ici avec plein de billets" (76).[3] Eventually, Djiraël and his family travel to the village where his father's funeral will be held; here, the culture shock is much greater than in Dakar. The funeral rites have many Senegalese traditions that often confuse Djiraël. He is, in fact, quite resistant to many aspects of the funeral and, by extension, mourning his father. One night, his aunt and mother come to see him and explain that he has one last chance to come to terms with his father's absence and death: "il faut que tu te rendes dans la forêt. Tu marcheras jusqu'à ce que tu repères l'endroit idéal pour méditer. Une fois que tu l'auras trouvé, tu t'assiseras seul et tu ne penseras qu'à ton père. Si tu te libères de toi-même, l'Harmattan t'apportera un message" (122).[4] The implication is that Djiraël's liberation from himself would truly be a liberation from his French identity: he could finally connect more fully with his African heritage.

Djiraël doesn't trust in any of these traditional beliefs, but sets out nonetheless. In the forest, he encounters a mystic old man who tells him a long, fairy tale-esque story of two lovers, Kadiom and Maléguène. Djiraël also shares stories of his own father, a man who Djiraël knew better by his absence than by his presence—"un père fantome" (152).[5] The old man eventually reveals to Djiraël that he carries a message from his father: that his father loved him. Djiraël is finally able to respond that he loved his father, too. Like *Un Papillon dans la Cité*, *Sarcelles-Dakar* is ultimately a hopeful story. Without diminishing the difficulties faced by Djiraël and Félicie, the two stories stress both the need for, and the possibility of, belonging.

[2] "Familiarize [himself] again with the neighborhood."

[3] "A little Senegalese from France who shows up loaded with cash."

[4] "You must enter the forest. You will walk until you find the ideal spot to meditate. Once you have found it, you will sit by yourself and think of nothing but your father. If you can free yourself, the Harmattan will bring you a message."

[5] "A ghost father."

Achieved Indigeneity: Hybridity in Coming-of-Age Identity Construction

The sense of belonging achieved by Djiraël and Félicie is not stagnant; their paths are not moving linearly toward a single, defined point. Instead, each protagonist achieves what Mimi Sheller describes as "an achieved indigeneity—a new claim of belonging to a locale, but a belonging *grounded in movement*, difference and transformation rather than stasis or permanence" (276, emphasis mine). This seemingly paradoxical idea—grounded movement—is an apt descriptor for the challenges faced by young adult migrant protagonists. Lafuente, too, highlights this process in young adult Caribbean-American literature, though I believe it can apply to any national or cultural migration context: "Thus, while the main characters are experiencing the personal journey of maturing from children to adults, they also undergo a literal journey in which they immigrate to the United States, where they develop hybrid identities as bicultural young adults" (34). Indeed, one of the hallmarks of maturation is learning to be independent from one's family, and finding one's place in a larger societal totality. Yet, within the migration narrative, leaving one's family often also represents leaving behind a significant portion of one's culture and former identity: becoming other. The paradoxical desire for independence and connection is typical of young adult novels, as well as in novels of migration; thus, when the two themes overlap, the effect is dramatically magnified.

This is particularly true of Félicie's story. In joining her mother in Paris, Félicie is simultaneously leaving home and going home. Aurélie writes to her, saying "Depuis mon départ, j'ai pensé à toi chaque jour … il est temps maintenant de me rejoindre en France où ta famille t'attend" (9).[6] Similarly, Félicie admits, "dans ma tête, j'avais déjà pris au moins mille fois l'avion" (15).[7] This is an expected reunification of daughter to mother, and citizen to motherland. Yet, despite imagining this meeting, all of Félicie's physical ties are firmly rooted in Guadeloupe—its culture, its landscapes, and the maternal familiarity of Man Ya. Thus, rather than navigating a simplistic duality—the safety of home versus the

[6] "Since leaving, I have thought about you every day… now, it is time for you to join me in France, where your family awaits."

[7] In my mind, I had already taken the flight at least a thousand times."

unknown—Félicie exists in a liminal space between the two, belonging to both and neither Man Ya and/nor Aurélie, Guadeloupe and/nor France.

Even once she is in Paris, her mother lives on the tenth floor of a towering apartment building, where Félicie has "l'impression d'être toujours dans l'avion, en suspens entre ciel et terre" (36).[8] The reimagined airplane serves to reinforce Félicie's disconnect from both her past and present realities; she hovers between the two, unable to fully embody either. Here, Félicie reflects Homi Bhabha's notion of a "third space," defined by Arup Ratan Chakraborty as "a place of opportunity for the growth of fresh ideas … it rejects anything fixed, so it opens up newer scope for fresh thoughts allowing us to go beyond the rigidity and limited focus of colonial binary thinking" (149). Chakraborty further elaborates on Bhabha's idea of hybridity: "the idea that no culture is really pure as it is always in contact with the other. According to [Bhabha], Hybridization is an ongoing process; it, therefore, cannot be 'still'" (149). Félicie is literally in motion, imagining herself on an airplane in between two homes; she remains suspended between Guadeloupe and France, connected to both, and rooted in neither.

From this vantage point, Félicie comes to embody one of the key French Caribbean literary figures identified by J. Michael Dash: the storyteller, "who occupies the literary foreground, with his insights into the group unconscious" (164). The storyteller figure suggests a sense of polyphony and hybridization; Félicie admits to her friend Mo that she keeps a notebook and writes down everything that happens to her. In this way, she records not only her own story, but those of her family and friends—seeking to understand and synthesize the stories of others with her own. The power of stories and the written word is undeniable in this book: from the Antillean Creole scattered throughout the text, to Félicie's mother writing to Man Ya for the first time in twenty years ("C'est grâce à notre Félicie que j'ai réalisé que la parole vaut mieux que toute forme de silence" [110]),[9] to author Gisèle Pineau's own childhood, spent growing up between Guadeloupe and France.

Un Papillon dans la Cité depicts the possibility of a cultural hybridity, maintaining an intangible connection to a larger diaspora while building a life in a new country. Kaisa Ilmonen observes that "in the European version [of the bildungsroman], the protagonist chooses, accepts and

[8] "The impression of still being in the plane, suspended between sky and earth."

[9] "It's thanks to our Félicie that I realized words are better than all forms of silence."

discards viewpoints or values on his way to a harmonious self" (72). In her identity development, Félicie's migration to France represents a literal, physical fragmentation between her roots in Guadeloupe and her mother in Paris. Unlike her European counterparts, however, Félicie *records* rather than discards the values and viewpoints of others as she circles between Guadeloupe and France. In this way, she does find a harmonious self as a storyteller—preserving the past and envisioning the future. Her time in France does not necessarily root her to the country, nor does she seek to become "French" to fit in. Rather, it pushes her to better understand her place in a larger, mobile diaspora whose members all experience the conflicting alienation and belonging of migration; in sharing their stories, she seeks to give a voice to this deeply personal yet universally fragmenting experience.

Like *Un Papillon dans la Cité*, Insa Sané's *Sarcelles-Dakar* contains some autobiographical elements. Born in 1974 in Dakar, Sané moved to France when he was only six years old to live in the Sarcelles suburb. Like his protagonist Djiraël, Sané also had to learn to exist between multiple cultures. Though he initially resisted his immersion into France, as an adult, he has a more optimistically nuanced view of his place in the world, explaining: "J'ai longtemps voulu croire que j'étais et resterai exclusivement Sénégalais, mais la vie m'a enseigné que je suis partout chez moi" (Sané, quoted in Idrisse).[10] In the beginning of *Sarcelles-Dakar*, Djiraël, too, tries to deny that living in France has impacted his identity; he believes himself to be an outsider in France—even as he speaks with Parisian slang and traverses the city with an easy confidence.

Once in Senegal, this fragmentation becomes a continuous source of frustration as his extended family mythologize his life in France. Djiraël begins to realize that he is deeply privileged in a way he has never before considered. This is the beginning of many uncomfortable challenges to Djiraël's fragile sense of self, which has been built between two cultures and two parents. It seems that he cannot get a grasp on either place; he simultaneously insists that he is Senegalese—*not* French—while also trying to prove that France is similar enough to Senegal that he understands life in Dakar. Thus, he has become simultaneously *other* by the French identity he resists and the Senegalese identity his family withholds. The

[10] "I have long wanted to believe that I was and would stay exclusively Senegalese, but life has taught me that I am at home everywhere."

impossibility of coalescing these ideas is a source of constant tension during his visit as he struggles to belong in both countries and even within his own family.

In fact, it is not only Djiraël's family who perceive him as a rich outsider. Later, when he goes shopping, he is quickly surrounded by a group of children begging: "Je ne parlais pas wolof mais je comprenais très bien qu'ils me demandaient de l'argent … putain, ça commençait sérieusement à me faire chier qu'on m'appelle francenabé" (84).[11] Djiraël's emotional response to these confrontations is typically defensive; despite his initial hesitation to travel to Senegal, it hurts him to feel ostracized from his home culture. At this point, Djiraël is still unable to accept a hybridized way of being: he oscillates between a conception of French *or* Senegalese, still believing that an identity must rest with one or the other.

His identity crisis reaches a turning point with his visit to the mystic storyteller in the forest. Here, his encounter is indicative of what Elodie Malanda calls the "esthétique du merveilleux" (312).[12] Before his message from the Harmattan, Djiraël scoffs at the idea of the supernatural, believing it to be mere superstition encouraged by his mother—an example of what Malanda calls Djiraël's European rationality. However, after his meeting in the forest, he recognizes that he has undergone a real, yet unquantifiable, experience, which signals:

> La victoire de la magie sur la logique rationaliste de l'Occident… [il doit] se rendre à l'évidence que le monde surnaturel existe, preuves à l'appui, une fois [qu'il est] de retour dans [son] pays natal. Le cartésianisme acquis en France y est alors présenté comme aliénant et la connexion [qu'il renoue] avec le monde surnaturel marque la fin d'une quête identitaire. (418)[13]

Thus, Djiraël comes to understand another way he has internalized a French identity; by reconnecting with Senegal, he is able to understand another way of looking at the world. His time with the Harmattan reconnects him to a larger Senegalese system of belief and cultural traditions

[11] "I didn't speak Wolof, but I clearly understood that they were asking me for money. Damn, it was starting to seriously piss me off that they called me francenabé!"

[12] "Aesthetic of the marvelous."

[13] "The triumph of magic over the rationalist logic of the West … he must acknowledge that the supernatural world exists, with supporting evidence, once he is back in his native country. The Cartesianism acquired in France is thus presented as alienating, and the connection that he renews with the supernatural world marks the end of an identity quest."

that he had inadvertently lost. A renewed spirituality is another layer in Djiraël's increasingly complex sense of self.

Djiraël's journey is also represented in the physical world as he loses or gives up some of the material things tying him to his life and status in Paris. In one scene, for example, as a part of a purification process during his father's funeral rites, he must shave his head. He is horrified: "merde. J'allais perdre ma belle coupe afro, que j'avais mis deux ans à faire pousser..." (116).[14] Yet it is this newfound baldness that allows him to once again feel the wind on his head—a clear foreshadowing to the coming Harmattan and his reconnection with his father. Furthermore, when he first arrives in Dakar, his cousins are jealous of his name brand shoes and clothes. At the end of the novel, his cousin begs for his shoes. Earlier in the story, for similar comments, Djiraël reacted with anger. Now, he can laugh: "voilà comment mes Air Max toutes neuves sont restées au bled... Plus de short Lacoste, plus de baskets Jordan et plus de tee-shirt Nike" (172–173).[15] Here, Djiraël symbolically demonstrates a deeper understanding of his own hybridity—he easily sheds the physical markers that he previously clung to, acknowledging their impermanence. Furthermore, he can recognize that the clothes have a different meaning and context for his cousins—one which Djiraël cannot fully experience.

In both *Un Papillon dans la Cité* and *Sarcelles-Dakar*, neither protagonist develops a stagnant identity. Their journeys toward adulthood in the context of migration necessitate a complex reimagining of belonging that embodies multiple geopolitical realities. Internalized ideas about France are reconstructed alongside their understanding of their own selves. By recognizing the (in)validity of the myth of France, Félicie and Djiraël are able to integrate their French experiences into their multifaceted identities. Each learns to cherish and nurture the connections they have with a multitude of cultures and places, thereby participating in Bhabha's ongoing process of hybridization.

[14] "I was going to lose my beautiful afro, the one I'd spent two years growing out...."

[15] "That's how my brand new Air Maxes stayed in the village ... No more Lacoste shorts, Jordan sneakers, or Nike tee-shirts."

Generational Power Structures: Influence and Impact

One further similarity between both *Un Papillon dans la Cité* and *Sarcelles-Dakar* is common to young adult literature in general: the protagonists' lack of agency (mirroring, in this case, the similar power imbalance between France and its former colonial holdings). Félicie and Djiraël are sent to and from France at the behest of their parents. In each case, the myth of a better life in France originates with the parental figures; it is up to each protagonist, then, to develop their own relationship with the country. This phenomenon is explored explicitly in Ilmonen's discussion of mothers and daughters in female French Caribbean writers, though the effect is felt in both novels: "It is particularly common to describe the problematic relationship between mother and daughter as a metaphor for the relationship between the colony and the colonized. The mother may be imbued with white ideals or too deeply wounded by them to teach her daughter any means of resistance" (69). Thus, Félicie and Djiraël work toward developing not only a sense of independence from the family unit, but also a separation from inherited ideals of colonization. Their coming-of-age is interconnected with their countries' parallel postcolonial identity development.

In *Un Papillon dans la Cité*, parental expectations and connections are explored through Félicie's own situation, as well as through observations of her friend's North African immigrant family. Mohamed Ben Doussan (nicknamed Mo) moved to France when he was five. In some ways, his family is different: Félicie's mother has married Papa Jo, has a job, and strives to forget Guadeloupe as she works to fit in with French society. Mo's mother and aunts, on the other hand, "ne trouvent pas de travail, ni d'mari … alors, elles mangent toute la journée des loukoums et des makroudes avec ma grande-mère en parlant du pays" (59).[16] Here again, Mo's experience is both known and unknown to Félicie; though they are both immigrants in the same Parisian apartment building, Mo's experiences are uniquely his own.

His story does, however, parallel with Félicie's in some explicit ways. Like Félicie, his strongest connection to his home country is through his grandmother, Fathia. On one visit, Fathia bakes loukoums for the

[16] "find neither work nor husbands … so they spend all day eating loukoums and makroudes with my grandmother, reminiscing about their country."

children. This sweet cake reminds Félicie of the doukouns Man Ya used to make, and she notes that: "Loukoum et doukoun, ça se joue sur la même musique, ça rime, c'est parent" (56).[17] Once again, there is a sense that Félicie's story is not strictly unidimensional; instead, it mirrors Mo's. Through "la même musique," we can see the multiplicity of Félicie's identity, as she finds common ground with other immigrants. Here, too, grandmothers—or elders in general—represent a wealth of heritage. Pineau seems to warn, however, that this cultural knowledge is impermanent; indeed, Félicie's presence in France instead of Guadeloupe reifies her physical separation from Man Ya. On another visit, Mo shows off a kouka in their apartment: "regarde celle-ci … C'est seulement ma grand-mère Fathia qui pourra te traduire les inscriptions" (59).[18] Even within one or two generations, then, traditions can begin to fade; it is up to the younger generations to try to preserve them.

Yet in this preservation, there is inevitably a loss and fragmentation as each subsequent generation passes on an inherently incomplete understanding. For Mo, Fathia embodies an explicit, whole identity, inextricable from her home country. However, she, too, is separated from her roots—while also bearing the burden of remembering and preserving her home culture. The knowledge she has is reduced to a few treasured artifacts, and memories that she creates and shares with Mo. Mo's perceptions of his home country, then, are necessarily partial—filtered through the eyes of another.

Despite their limitations, these matrilineal connections are typical of literature from the Caribbean and integral to identity development. Ilmonen writes about the important role grandmothers play in the Caribbean bildungsroman: "the grandmother characters are constructed via a genealogy of feminist resistance and Caribbean women's cultural tradition…As part of her growth, the daughter or granddaughter must seek out her matrilinear tradition" (69). Once discovered, the daughter or granddaughter can begin to reconnect with the motherland. The motherland here is not a physical space; it is rather "a mutual relationship between a diasporic people that emphasizes continuity, camaraderie and communality. In Caribbean women's writing, the finding of such a matrilinear and folkloric connection to the collective tradition is a particular form of the postcolonial bildung quest" (69). Thus, Félicie and Mo can gain a sense of

[17] "Loukoum and doukoun, they play the same music, they rhyme, they're kindred."
[18] "look at this one … only my grandmother Fathia can translate the inscriptions for you."

belonging through their grandmothers, even if they are physically in France. The kouka in Mo's apartment, then, represents the possibility of learning to read the inscriptions and becoming connected to a diaspora larger than himself. Together, Mo and Félicie represent a new generation—it is up to them to remember their ancestry while building an identity that is their own, even if their "own" self has elements of "fragmentation and friction between … different axes of identity" (Ilmonen 72).

This process is similar, yet subverted, in *Sarcelles-Dakar*, though the focus is more concentrated on Djiraël's paternal connections, symbolized through his spiritual walk in the woods to meet the Harmattan—winds that could carry a message from his father. Again, this both echoes and contrasts *Un Papillon dans la Cité*; both are about absent parents. However, while Félicie's relationship with her mother was damaged, they could work together to repair it and let something new flourish. For Djiraël, the opportunity has passed, and he can only hope to find closure with his father—and by extension, better understand his relationship to Senegal. This is mirrored in the fable told by the old man in the woods about two lovers who must, for reasons beyond their control, be separated for a long time. It is only when they are reunited that they find peace. Of course, the story evokes Djiraël's own bitter separation from his father and homeland. It is only when Djiraël is able to tell the old man in the woods, "Dites-lui … que je l'aime également et que … je suis fier d'être son fils" (166),[19] that he is able to move forward without resentment. While he is talking about his father, the moment also clearly evokes his evolved attitude toward Senegal. He had long felt Senegalese without fully confronting what that part of his identity meant. It is only in reuniting with his father's ghostly messenger, in his home country, that Djiraël can begin to reconcile his past, present, and future.

Yet he has also not entirely embraced the faith espoused by his mother and aunts; he doesn't quite believe that anything supernatural happened in the forest, for example. Perhaps unconsciously still adhering to Western notions of individualism, he explains,

> Les esprits des morts ne pouvaient pas communiquer avec les vivants. Les contes, c'était pour les enfants, et la foi pour les faibles. En réalité, le vrai problème, avant ma rencontre avec Kadiom, c'est que j'avais perdu la foi. J'avais d'abord arrêté de croire en l'amour de mon père. Ensuite, j'avais

[19] "Tell him … that I love him too and that … I'm proud to be his son."

> cessé de croire en moi. Et puis, j'avais fini par ne plus croire en rien ni en personne. (173)[20]

In a nod to a newfound sense of community, however, Djiraël's new outlook is based on the intangible relationships he has with others—his father, his family, and a larger network of his ancestors. Most importantly, he has rekindled a sense of faith in himself; in this way he is able to be, as Sané said, "partout chez lui."[21] Fascinatingly, the novel never explicitly clarifies what happens in the forest, and readers are left to wonder if they can trust Djiraël's insistence that nothing supernatural occurred. Thus, the novel itself becomes a site of unshareable knowledge between author, narrator, and reader, reinforcing Djiraël's journey toward finding a sense of meaning in his own embodied experiences.

Djiraël's story is distinctly similar to Félicie's; both have aspects of their identities tied up in their relationships with their parents. This is a common theme in young adult literature, where the adolescent's growing independence outside of the family home is a hallmark of coming-of-age stories. Yet Djiraël and Félicie also have the added element of migration, complicating their search for identity. In both cases, they must explore what it means to leave the home—physically, emotionally, and culturally. For Djiraël, growing away from his father also pushed him to unconsciously grow away from Senegal. For Félicie, reconnecting with her mother put her in the uncomfortable position of losing the stability of her other maternal figure, Man Ya; without the anchor of Guadeloupe, Félicie became unrooted. In the end, too, both have better understandings of themselves as separate from their parents—which they are paradoxically only able to achieve through (physically or spiritually) *rejoining* their parents.

[20] The spirits of the dead could not communicate with the living. Stories are for children, faith for the weak. In reality, the real problem is that before my meeting with Kadiom, I had lost faith. I had first stopped believing in the love of my father. Then, I had stopped believing in myself. And then, I ended up not believing in anything or anyone.

[21] "At home everywhere."

Linguistic Hybridity in Transnational Spaces

Even within a French young adult text, there is a sense of hybridity in both the language and setting. Both Félicie and Djiraël navigate their roots within the Parisian banlieues—transnational spaces that allow them to connect with other immigrants. Living in a multicultural space pushes them to what Bhabha describes as the "gathering of exiles and émigrés and refugees; gathering on the edge of 'foreign' cultures; gathering at frontiers; gathering in the ghettos or cafes of city centers" (Bhabha, quoted in Chakraborty, 150). Here, on the edges of Paris—at the frontier of the de facto cultural center of France—Djiraël and Félicie live in their own multilingual and multicultural microcosms. Like Félicie's polyphony, Djiraël's journey between Senegal and France shows him the multiplicity of his own identity. In *Sarcelles-Dakar* and *Un Papillon dans la Cité*, Djiraël and Félicie exist in a liminal space between French culture and their home culture communities, embodying new, transformational identities that move beyond colonial binary thinking. France is a physical home for them while they simultaneously thrive in the multiplicity of larger diasporas.

This is reflected linguistically in both novels; each story directly juxtaposes formal French written-language hegemony with elements of local languages and vernaculars. *Un Papillon dans la Cité*, for example, frequently includes words or phrases in Antillean Creole, which are always translated with footnotes at the bottom of the page. The inclusion of Creole is in line with what Dash describes as "a new literary multilingualism that combines French and Creole," representing "an epistemological break with previous French Caribbean writing" (164). For Dash, the hybridization of language is part of an "earlier vitality" returning to the literature of the region, as well as a symbolic "widespread questioning of the notions of authenticity and 'enracinement'" (163–164). He further goes on to note that Caribbean writing need not be produced in the Caribbean; the Caribbean diaspora (including Pineau, herself born in Paris to Guadeloupian parents) now produces works across the world. Thus, structurally, the book mimics Félicie herself, as she becomes a global citizen embodying a new type of linguistic and cultural hybridity.

Where *Un Papillon dans la Cité* was infused with Antillean Creole, *Sarcelles-Dakar* is notable for its distinctly Parisian *argot*. The novel opens with a single exclamation: "Putain!"[22] followed by a jargon-filled

[22] "Fuck!"

conversation between Djiraël and his friend Armand. Djiraël's first person narration is equally distinctive throughout the novel. For example, he describes getting ready before going out: "Une putain de douche bien chaude! Ça c'est un de mes kiffes" (17).[23] Djiraël's narration anchors the book to the outskirts of Paris, whereas *Un Papillon dans la Cité* remains tied to Guadeloupe and the Caribbean. For Félicie, Creole is a way to stay connected to her home country, but also to express a linguistic hybridity in French Caribbean literature, tying her to a larger tradition of storytellers.

Language has a similar function in *Sarcelles-Dakar*. It is, as noted by Malanda, a way for Sané to:

> s'inscri[re] dans ce que Bernard Mouralis définit comme "contre-littérature", c'est-à-dire les écrits qui éclatent les limites de ce qui est considéré comme de la "littérature." Cette contestation depuis la marge—ici sociale—est soulignée à travers l'alternance de chapitres entièrement écrits dans la langue "des cités" … Sané montre ici que tous les langages sociaux ont leur place dans la littérature. (312)[24]

Djiraël's *argot*, then, is transformed from a marginalized dialect into a valid, hybridized way of speaking that ties him to a larger Parisian community. However, it is also an (unconscious) marker of Djiraël's distance from his home country—a separation that he spends the rest of the book navigating. Ultimately, as Bhabha theorizes, neither Félicie nor Djiraël has a "still" identity. Linguistically, they embody a multitude of distinct partialities that ultimately coalesce into singular, vibrant identities. Their cultural hybridization—connecting elements of French, Creole, Parisian, Senegalese, and more—is a constant negotiation and renegotiation between a plurality of places, people, languages, and traditions.

[23] "A hot fucking shower. That's the shit."

[24] "be a part of what Bernard Mouralis defines as 'counter-literature,' or writing that breaks the limits of what is considered to be 'literature.' This contestation from the margins—in this case, social ones—is highlighted through the alternation of chapters written entirely in the language of 'the cities.' Sané demonstrates that all social languages have their place in literature."

Conclusion

Un Papillon dans la Cité and *Sarcelles-Dakar* both explore the dynamics of growing up across multiple cultures and countries. Their protagonists are admirably resilient, adapting to the constant demands and expectations of their families, friends, and internalized assumptions. The Parisian banlieues, an important setting in both novels, create a fascinating backdrop against which Félicie and Djiraël navigate their roles in diverse global diasporas. In this chapter, I have attempted to demonstrate that these young adult narratives of migration represent a fascinating intersection of two literary traditions, enriching the exploration of identity construction. Despite their depth, however, young adult literature and its varied subgenres are often overlooked among the broader critical scholarship. Indeed, the genre is often critiqued as unworthy of consideration among adult readers and academics; Karen Coats notes that young adult literature often falls outside of the "literary," being labeled instead as popular or pedagogical (389).

Through *Un Papillon dans la Cité* and *Sarcelles-Dakar*, I argue that this is an unfortunate misconception. In these novels, the challenges of migration both complement and transform the traditional developmental passage to adulthood, necessitating new, hybridized identity constructions. Modern young adult novels have the capacity to tackle intricate global and societal issues, while simultaneously exploring the complex inner lives of their adolescent protagonists. Though this chapter focused on role of France, the stories fit into a larger narrative of growing up in a geopolitically unstable and fragmented world. The delicacy with which these novels are able to portray this identity fragmentation is a testament to the genre's legitimacy. Young adult literature is thus a rich source for scholarly analysis, defying a tendency to relegate it to the periphery of literary academia.

Bibliography

Chakraborty, Arup Ratan. "Liminality in Post-Colonial Theory: A Journey from Arnold van Gennep to Homi K. Bhabha." *Anadhyun: An International Journal of Social Sciences* (AIJSS), vol. 1, no. 1, 2016, pp. 145–53.

Chambers, Aidan. "Finding the Form: Towards a Poetics of Youth Literature." *The Lion and the Unicorn*, vol. 34, 2010, pp. 267–283.

Coats, Karen. "Conventions of Children's Literature: Then and Now." *Style*, vol. 35, no. 3, 2001, pp. 389–392.

Dash, J. Michael. "Textual Error and Cultural Crossing: A Caribbean Poetics of Creolization." *Research in African Literatures*, vol. 25, no. 2, 1994, pp. 159–168.

Fanon, Frantz. *Peau noire, masques blancs*. Editions de Seuil, 1952.

Idrisse, Irène. "Transfigurateur du réel: Insa Sané, écrivain et slameur." *Le Petit Journal*, 17 April 2018, https://lepetitjournal.com/dakar/communaute/transfigurateur-du-reel-insa-sane-ecrivain-et-slameur-228437.

Ilmonen, Kaisa. "Talking Back to the Bildungsroman." *Journal of West Indian Literature*, vol. 25, no. 1, 2017, pp. 60–76.

Lafuente, Elia Michelle. "Nationhood, Struggle, and Identity." *Contemporary Adolescent Literature and Culture*: The Emergent Adult, edited by Maria Nikolajeva and Mary Hilton, Taylor & Francis Group, 2012, pp. 33–45.

Lesne, Élisabeth. "Omar Ba, Je suis venu, j'ai vu, je n'y crois plus." *Hommes & Migrations*, 2009, pp. 206–207.

Malanda, *Elodie. L'Afrique dans les romans pour la jeunesse en France et en Allemagne 1991–2010*. Éditions Champion, 2019.

Pineau, Gisèle. *Un Papillon dans la Cité*. Éditions Sepia, 1992.

Sané, Insa. *Sarcelles-Dakar*. Sarbacane, 2009.

Sheller, Mimi. "Creolization in Discourses of Global Culture." *Uprootings / Regroupings*, edited by Sara Ahmed, Claudia Castaneda, Anne-Marie Fortier, and Mimi Sheller, Routledge, 2020.

Making the Rounds: Information, Belief, and Breath in Alice Walker's "Strong Horse Tea"

Jodi Cressman

I used to think that there would one day be a vaccine: that if enough black people named the virus, explained it, demonstrated how it operates, videoed its effects, protested it peacefully, revealed how widespread it really is, how the symptoms arise, how so many Americans keep giving it to each other, irresponsibly and shamefully, generation after generation, causing intolerable and unending damage both to individual bodies and to the body politic—I thought if that knowledge became as widespread as could possibly be managed or imagined that we might finally reach some kind of herd immunity. I don't think that anymore.

—Zadie Smith, *from "Intimations"*

J. Cressman (✉)
Dominican University, River Forest, IL, USA
e-mail: jcressman@dom.edu

J. Cressman et al. (eds.), *Envisioning Embodiment in the Health Humanities*, Sustainable Development Goals Series,
https://doi.org/10.1007/978-3-031-49807-7_10

Introduction: Reading and Breathing

Written in the first year of the COVID pandemic, Smith's "Intimations" likens the operations of contempt—specifically of racism and economic violence—to the virus shuttering communities and overwhelming hospital corridors with patients gasping for air. As we all now know, the COVID vaccine, which would arrive within a year of Smith's essay, mitigated the spread and damage of the virus but failed to secure herd immunity. Vaccine refusal was less attributable to gaps in information, which was in wide circulation, than to gaps in belief, as scientific narratives circulated among other stories about the virus: it was a hoax, it was similar to the flu, it was less dangerous than the vaccine itself. Smith observes that access to knowledge, for similar reasons, is insufficient for dismantling racism and poverty; however widely circulated, hard data and even "ocular proof" don't inoculate against racist contempt. Still, even if Smith no longer believes that information can lead to immunity from racist contempt, she must nonetheless believe in sustained if localized efforts at mitigation. Bringing visibility to insidious and implicit beliefs can lead to material action and systemic transformation: otherwise, why write?

This chapter attempts a response to that question—why write?—as central to the work of the critical medical humanities, worthy of inclusion on the list of questions that Jo Winning has identified as forming the field: "What is a body? What are its boundaries and its contours? Can we ever really know the body in its entirety, or only ever in its parts? How do we come to know the body through the senses? And what does it mean to be a body and to encounter the body of the Other?" (325). Winning's final question here, with its focus on the body of an "Other" that may not only be sick, but is also gendered and racialized, offers a useful lens for intersectional approaches to studies of embodiment and the health humanities. Bodies can be threatened and can be misread as threatening; they can be vulnerable to infection and can also be racially coded as infectious. Winning's question is also useful in the way it turns the lens on the body doing the encountering, whether that may be a body of the clinician, a white body, a male body. As Winning goes on to explain, it is the clinician's body, and not just the patient's, that "might similarly be made docile and have lost its ability to utilise all of its sensorium" (330). In other words, the critical medical humanities might benefit by studying the inherently incomplete, embodied experiences of the person who is quite literally "making sense" of the Other who is in pain or suffering.

I am principally concerned with the entanglement of that sense-making—that is, the circulation of information that constitutes reading (and misreading), whether a text or the body of the Other—and the circulation (and blockage) of breath. Similar to Zadie Smith, the Afro-Latina poet Yesenia Montilla overlays the COVID virus that was interfering with breathing onto the murders of Black men who had been misread as threats by the police who choked them to death. The speaker of Montilla's "a brief meditation of breath" yokes them together, noting that

> the last time i'd think of death with breath / was that balmy day in july when the cops /became a raging fire & sucked the breath / out of Garner; but yesterday i walked/ 38 blocks to my father's house with a mask / over my nose & mouth, the sweat dripping / off my chin only to get caught in fabric & pool up / like rain.

Just as police are, ostensibly, anyway, the remedy for crime, they can also be its perpetrators, here figured as a fiery vacuum, "suck[ing] the breath out of Garner," while both COVID and its preventive mask are blocking the circulation of breath in the speaker, the products of her own body (the sweat) pooling "like rain" in her mask and obstructing the flow of air. The poem's short, regular lines make visible—in fact, in the reader, make *palpable*—the regularity of breathing. The line breaks further draw attention to broken, labored breath, pointing to the gap between "sucked the breath" and "out of Garner." The breathlessness at the heart of the poem is, in this way, literally transmitted from the body of the poem's speaker to its reader, emphasizing the capacity of both breathing and reading to bridge the inner and exterior worlds.

The poem ends on an abrupt note, linking the bodies whose lives ended too soon, with the body of the poem that remains, perpetually, unfinished:

> they say it's so contagious it could be quite
> breathtaking. so persistent it might as well
> be breathing down your neck—

The contagious "it" in Montilla's poem, which can be traced syntactically to both the coronavirus and racist contempt, is breathtaking in the sense of literally overawing the senses and reason, but also in the sense of overtaking the body, "breathing down your neck." The victim of suffocation, here at the poem's end, has shifted from the speaker who struggled to walk in a mask and from Eric Garner, mentioned earlier by name, outside of the boundaries of the poem: it is now *you*, the reader. The black space within the final line points to the cessation of both speech and breath, as it is literally unspeakable, marked in a verbal reading by silence, and the final dash signals a conclusive break, with the unspoken words that might follow being pointed to but never brought into the shared world.

Like Smith's essay, Montilla's poem presents literature as a kind of imaging technology that can shed light and render form, if only by pointing, to the otherwise invisible acts of breathing and reading that mediate the interior and exterior worlds (McNaughton and Carel). In this way, the literary text becomes a tool at our disposal, especially in the extra-clinical space of public health, as it illuminates the entanglements and disrupted circuitries of the body, language, illness, and death.

Taking on this book's concern with information and embodied experiences as a snarl of partialities and segments that are synthesized into larger, meaningful wholes, this chapter explores the incomplete circuits and segments at the heart of Alice Walker's short story, "Strong Horse Tea," published about fifty years before Montilla's poem and Smith's essay about the viral patterns linking COVID to racist contempt, but sharing their central concerns. The story follows the plight of Rannie, desperate to get suitable medical care for her infant Snooks, who is dying from an infectious respiratory illness, described in the story as whooping cough or pneumonia. The circulation of Snooks's breath has been disrupted by his illness, but that is just one of the many incomplete circuits in the story. Rannie's illiteracy creates a gap in the circulation of written information found in newspaper flyers and her mailman's racism creates a gap in the circulation of spoken information, as he neither correctly receives nor fully transmits her request for medical help. Once she accepts the reality that the help she requested will not arrive, Rannie resorts to the medical advice of her granny doctor neighbor to retrieve horse urine from a neighboring farm; however, Snooks has died before she's able to administer the dose, a fact that the reader but not Rannie herself knows.

"Strong Horse Tea" was published 1973, but is set around fifty years or so earlier in Jim Crow South in the decades of legal racial segregation, expansion of germ theory, a widely promised but mostly undelivered access to public health, and the widespread implementation of free rural mail delivery. Whereas Trudier Harris and other seminal scholars working on Black women writers have focused on the vertical or diachronic gaps at the work in the story—that is, Rannie's break with matrilineage and folk medicine—this chapter looks at the synchronic gaps in the multiple circuits of meaning in the story. My analysis situates the two primary (and broken) circuits in the story—breathing and information—within historical context, highlighting the ways that bodies are "read" through cultural and racialized lenses and, further, the way that reading itself is an embodied practice. In fact, I argue, the story seems to end in the reader's body, as a kind of pause between breaths, making visible the gap between knowledge and action.

Beyond pointing to the systemic inequalities in access to modern medicine, "Strong Horse Tea" suggests the ways that "folk" and "modern" medicine are overlapping practices, with each grounded in "unscientific" beliefs. In his important work on medical racism, John Hoberman has argued that all of the knowledge of facts and statistics about disparities in health outcomes hasn't led to any meaningful change in practice. The facts remain in an "abstract dimension untethered to living human experience" (5). The study of literature, undertaken as part of efforts in the wider health humanities, can partly restore that broken tether, connecting abstract statistics to particular, human stories. Given the ambiguity of its ending, the "message" of Walker's story is, like the mailman's, never fully delivered from writer to reader; rather, its meaning points to a gap, calling for response.

Folk Medicine and Belief in "Strong Horse Tea"

At the emotional heart of Alice Walker's short story "Strong Horse Tea" (1973) is the baby Snooks, who tragically dies of whooping cough and/or double pneumonia, despite his mother Rannie's desperate attempts to save him, first by rejecting and then ultimately accepting the "folk medicine" prescribed by her older neighbor Sarah. But the actual center of the story—its middle section, which abruptly moves the focus to an event that takes place earlier in the day and outside the rural cabin where Snooks lies dying—documents Rannie's interaction with her mailman.

At first, the narrative intrusion is jarring, until one recognizes it as merely one of many ruptures or blockages throughout the text. Snooks is dying because air cannot circulate through his compromised lungs; the mailman never delivers Rannie's message to the town's (white) doctor; similarly, Rannie does not deliver the "horse tea" she collects from the pasture to its intended recipient; Rannie's initial rejection of Sarah's treatment suggests a generational break in cultural practices; the words in the newspaper delivered to Rannie by the mailman never complete a circuit of meaning because of her illiteracy; and the circulation of air through her cabin walls is itself blocked by those same unread newspapers, newly repurposed as insulation.

Much of the critical attention on this story has zeroed in on Rannie's initial rejection of folk medicine, reading Snooks's death as a corrective to her dismissal of her cultural inheritance; however, as I argue, the text's extensive focus on broken circuits –in healthcare, the economy, information, and in the body—suggests that we should instead interpret the meaning of the "strong horse tea" and the larger practice of folk medicine in context of the wider systems circulating—or failing to circulate—in and beyond the text. Sarah's "alternative medicine" is not one choice among many; in fact, it is not actually an "alternative" at all—it is Rannie's only option in light of the pervasive medical racism that blocked access to modern medicine in the Jim Crow South. The responsibility for Snooks's death does not reside in a single person—Rannie, Sarah, or even the mailman, though he surely is the most culpable individual in the story—but is a failure of multiple economic, informational, and healthcare systems.

The meaning of the story itself never really comes "full circle." The ending points to one more information gap, as the reader knows that Snooks has already died but the final sentence depicts Rannie running home to give him "the still warm tea" (98). The ending could be interpreted as an example of ambivalence that is both archetypically literary and ultimately inert, but its attention to the gap between knowing and acting could be—and, I argue, should be –instead read as a call for political change. John Hoberman, among others, has pointed to the chasm between the abundant statistical documentation of disparities in medical care for Black and white Americans and meaningful, systemic, and sustained efforts to address them (5). Walker's story, like other works within the wider arts and health humanities field, contextualizes a well-known statistical reality within a representation of a human, embodied experience, urging us to close the gap in health access and outcomes.

While much of Walker's story depicts the generational conflict between the two women, the work is also concerned with communication pathways and, specifically, the circuit of information that would *in theory* allow Rannie access to what she calls a "REAL doctor" practicing modern medicine as well as the racial bias that *in practice* breaks that circuit and prevents Snooks from receiving the mainstream antibacterial agents newly in use to treat pneumonia in the middle of the last century (Podolsky). In addition to Rannie and Sarah, the key figure "making the rounds" in this story does not even practice medicine. The mailman, who remains nameless because it is his function rather than his particularity that matters most, tells Rannie that "we'll do what we can" (92), but since he filters Rannie's request through racist stereotypes, he fails to grasp the gravity of Snooks's situation and takes the urgent message only to Sarah, who lives in the next house on his rural route.

Walker's story takes place in the mid-twentieth century, a time of promised transformation in health care, as historian Karen Kruse Thomas has documented, with the U.S. Public Health Service committing to improvements in services for rural, Southern African-Americans. Thomas Parran, who served as the sixth Surgeon General of the United States from 1936 to 1948, declared:

> [N]o one in the United States should be denied access to health and medical services because of economic status, race, geophysical location, or any other non-health factor of condition. It is a duty of governments—local, State, or Federal—to guarantee healthful living conditions and to enable every person to secure freedom from preventable disease. (Qtd. in Thomas 135)

However, despite his promise of equity, it was Parran who oversaw the notoriously racist Tuskegee syphilis experiment. Further, as Thomas points out, Parran's initiative that ostensibly aimed to serve African Americans resulted in a "deluxe Jim Crow" system that saw a vigorous construction of new hospitals and medical services that ultimately maintained segregation and structural inequities. Read in this historical context, the meaning of Walker's story becomes less about a binary choice between folk medicine and modern medicine and more a story about the overlapping economic, information, and health systems that simultaneously advertise and deny access.

Information and health systems are intertwined throughout the text, starting with Sarah's muttered chant that explains –or would explain, if Rannie could hear it—why her son will never get the treatment he needs: "White mailman, white doctor" (89). Additionally, as Deborah Anne Hooker points out, Snook's dying is closely connected to the newspaper circulars that the mailman brings, with the child's labored breathing sounding "like the wind pushing down damp papers in a shallow ditch" (89). Walker's yoking of information and health complicates the meaning of (and culpability for) Snooks's death, suggesting that he did not die because his mother initially rejected traditional medicine, nor even because of her illiteracy, in this case her failure to read the mailman's intentions. Instead, Walker points to the ironic and disastrous consequences of the *mailman*'s illiteracy—his inability to accurately decode her urgent message in the first place.

Rannie is functionally illiterate in the traditional sense, unable to read the newspaper circulars that the mailman delivers to her home. Though she cannot read the words on the advertisements, she is, ironically, able to note the absurdity in the system that keeps bringing them. As she says to the mailman, "She couldn't ever buy any of the things in the pictures—so why did the stores keep sending them to her?" (91). The advertisements are delivered, but cannot be read; this information breakdown is echoed in the broken economic system, as goods are produced and advertised to people too poor to afford them. Still, Rannie finds some use for the circulars as insulation to block drafts from her home. This irony—that the circulars find a use for Rannie in preventing circulation—echoes the paradox of the mailman failing to deliver a message to the correct address.

Rannie's illiteracy is rooted in geographical isolation and poverty; the mailman's more consequential illiteracy—his inability to properly "read" Rannie's situation—is rooted in racism. Just as Rannie can see the images in the circulars without being able to interpret them, the mailman hears her individual words but does not connect them together in meaningful ways, giving "little attention to what she was saying about her sick baby" and resenting her for letting the rain into his truck as she was "gabbing away about 'Snooks' and 'NEWmonia' and 'shots' and how she wanted a 'REAL doctor'" (91). It is not, the story makes clear, that he is idiosyncratically uncaring or cruel. He nods "sympathetically" (91) and takes care so as not "to hurt her feelings" (92). The root cause of his failure is his racism: "Black people as Black as Rannie Mae always made him uneasy, especially when they didn't smell good, and when you could tell they didn't right away" (91–92). His racism blocks Rannie's specific request for a doctor from being fully heard, as he immediately translates her words into the dead end of a stereotype: "Why did colored folks always want you to do something for them?" (92).

The mailman can't read Rannie's behavior, but neither can she "read through the lines" of his. When Sarah voices skepticism that the doctor will arrive, Rannie protests incredulously: "Who'd go and ignore a little sick baby like my Snooks?" (89). Sarah, however, knows that the doctor will never come and will, in fact, never get the message. "Some folks we don't know so well as we thinks we do might," she tells Rannie (89). Importantly, Sarah is both an expert in natural remedies and in reading—a "conjure woman" who has access to the hidden forces at work in nature and culture alike.

The mailman's circular travels from town to country and back, which should have kicked off a doctor's travel along the same route, is instead visually echoed by the path Rannie takes to the pasture to retrieve the mare's urine. Having no container with her, Rannie first collects the urine in her shoe and then, once the shoe leaks, she carries it in her mouth, running home to deliver it to her baby. However, baby Snooks had died in the meantime; several paragraphs before describing Rannie's return, the story notes that his "frail breathing had stopped with the thunder, not to come again" (97). In this case, as in her conversation with the mailman, the circuit is ultimately broken: neither the message nor the medicine arrives at its intended destination in time.

While home remedies, such as the one that Sarah offers to Rannie, might be commonly understood as a niche medical practice, they are actually by far the most widely practiced medical treatment in the United States (Harley 443). The traditional practice of African American folk medicine was informed both by the institution of slavery and a tangle of conflicting narratives about Black bodies and health. Some slaveowners permitted and even encouraged "granny doctors" to provide medical care for their enslaved population (Bronson and Nuriddon 714), at times because of the difficulty of finding a white doctor in geographically remote areas and, at other times, because of beliefs about biological differences between Black and white bodies. While the advent of germ theory in the mid-nineteenth century might have created wider understanding about the role of environmental factors in spreading contagious illnesses, it was instead powerfully contorted to "confirm" beliefs about the racial inferiority (and particular susceptibility) of Black bodies. These beliefs about a biological basis for African American inferiority led not only to blaming sick people for their illnesses and widespread concern among white physicians in the Jim Crow South about African Americans "infecting" white communities but also to ideas about an entire medical taxonomy of "Negro diseases" (Bronson and Nuriddon, 711). We can see the legacy of these beliefs in the mailman's belief that if Sarah's "magic ... didn't work on whites [it] probably would on Blacks" (92).

However, slaveowner attitudes about folk medicine were far from uniform, and some outright banned its practice. The common prohibition against home remedies in slavery meant that, as Bronson and Nuridden point out, indigenous practices of health care were means of expressing Black independence and resistance (715). In any case, regardless of whether folk remedies were encouraged or banned by slaveowners, it is unambiguously the case that slavery robbed enslaved people of their autonomy over their bodies and health.

The idea of folk medicine as a site of resistance will figure prominently in the critical reception of Walker's story. Much of the critical attention to Walker's story focuses on the ambiguity around Sarah's motivations for sending Rannie to the pasture for the horse urine. Does Sarah want to punish Rannie for her initial rejection of her cultural inheritance or does she earnestly believe in its curative powers? David Estes, for example, strongly argues for the latter interpretation. On the one hand, Estes sees Sarah's medicine as an intentionally oppositional practice that extends "a powerful tradition of resistance to white racism, a cultural reality she wants Rannie to accept" (221), but he also notes that "numerous folk beliefs held by African Americans attest to the powers of urine" (217). Interestingly, whatever the extent horse urine was used in traditional folk medicine at this time, it did play a role in modern medicine. Premarin, whose name derives from the words pregnant mare, was used as early as 1942 for treating hot flashes associated with menopause and, in the 1950s prednisone, a steroid found in horse urine, was commonly used to treat inflammatory diseases of the lung. In any case, for Estes, the story upholds Walker's admiration for African American's folk traditions, which she first learned through the anthropological research done by Zora Neale Hurston, to whom *In Love and Trouble* is dedicated.

Dellita Martin also sees the story's major conflict as between traditional forms of healing in African American culture and western medicine: "one wonders if the death of her baby is the price that Raney [sic] Toomer has to pay for rejecting her own culture. Unlike the first story, the value system of Black mythology is ineffective simply because the character no longer believes in it" (67). Like Estes and Martin, Trudier Harris reads the story as asserting the power—even the superiority—of folk medicine: "Walker does not view the folk culture as something separate from life, but as an integral and useful part of one's existence" (7). Even if Rannie is unable to save Snooks, Sarah's medicine reconnects her to a cultural tradition and history that might save her, especially in the wake of her impending grief. For Harris, Sarah's prescription of horse urine is "repulsive" and given that Sarah did not list it among her earlier suggestions for remedies, she may have the medicine as a punishment for Rannie for her earlier dismissal.

Each of these critics focuses on Rannie's break with tradition with her insistence on a "REAL doctor" and situates their reading of the text within the larger history of African American folk medicine as a powerful—possibly superior—model of healing. Harris suggests that the story points to the consequences of choosing the "white world" over one's own tradition and heritage, arguing that "Blacks can reject folk wisdom (Aunt Sarah) and the historical aspect of their heritage only by sacrificing something equally precious (Snooks, the son), a part of themselves" (7). In Harris's reading, Snooks's death is the price Rannie pays for rejecting her history and the practice of her ancestors. However, as a wider study of access to modern medicine in the Jim Crow South suggests, folk medicine was likely Rannie's only option for her son. Whether or not Rannie believed in it, she was shut out of access to modern medicine because of persistent beliefs among whites about the Black body.

Promise and Distrust: Access to Modern Medicine in the Jim Crow South

Just as Walker's text cannot be understood without a knowledge of folk medicine, any understanding of Rannie's distrust in folk medicine and Sarah's equally powerful (and ultimately justified) distrust of modern medicine equally depends on an understanding of both the innovations and moral bankruptcies in public health in the mid-twentieth century. Attending to the structural realities of access to healthcare (in whatever form) and access to health education sheds significant light on the material conditions of embodiment—that is, bodies circulate (or are blocked from circulation) in social conditions that facilitate or prevent care.

Rannie's initial rejection of folk medicine seems to stem from two entangled beliefs: that home remedies are ineffective (and possibly even harmful) and that modern medicine is both available and better. In rebuffing Sarah's initial attempts at help, Rannie "fiercely" retorts: "I don't believe in none of that swamp magic. All the home remedies I took when I was a child come just short of killing me" (88). What Rannie does believe in is the "magic bullet" of modern medicine. Her description of what she expects from the white doctor's "shots" echoes the hyperbolic language of the very advertisements she is unable to read: "We going to git some of them shots that makes peoples well, cures 'em of all they ails, cleans 'em out and makes 'em strong all at the same time" (90). In many ways, Rannie's belief in the magic bullet of the "shots that makes peoples well" was not unfounded. In 1927, pneumonia was the leading cause of death in the United States, but the development of anti-serums in the next decade would transform it from a top public health menace to a routine matter handled by private physicians (Podolsky). Even if Rannie could not read, she is likely to have heard the stories about these seemingly "magic" cures making the rounds, quite possibly from peddlers who, as an antecedent to the mailman's delivery of circulars, joined the practice of commerce with the spreading of information (often in the form of gossip).

Rannie might also have learned of the public health efforts that culminated in the Hill-Burton Act, which Truman signed into law in 1946. Hill-Burton brought significant construction of hospitals and health services, especially in the rural South. In return for the federal assistance, the hospitals could not discriminate on the basis of race. However, what Rannie may not have known (but what Sarah may have understood) is that these "biracial" hospitals housed segregated wards, as they were permitted to offer "separate but equal" treatment to their patients. The promise of modern medicine, together with the racist reality of its practice, helps explain both Rannie's excitement around the shots and Sarah's deep mistrust of white physicians. To be sure, this interpretation does not dispute Estes's and Harris's insistence on folk medicine as a valued and powerful tradition; rather, it suggests that Sarah's medical practice was not just an act of resistance, but also an historical necessity. While Estes is right to note that "'Strong Horse Tea' is set in the economically developed South where physicians now provide much of the health care," the literary and historical record suggests that these provisions were unequal at best (214).

While Estes argues that African Americans "lacked confidence in white medicine" in part because "it was not congruent with their traditional understanding of illness and its relationship to the spiritual realm of life," there were other reasons for Black to lack confidence in white physicians (218). In the middle of the last century, Black life expectancy had risen to 57 as opposed to 66 years for whites (Hoberman 19). Whites were (and still are) more likely to receive surgical treatment for heart disease and to be treated for pain (Hoberman 84) while Black bodies were more likely than white bodies to be objects for medical education (Bronson and Nuridden 709).

As the editor of the volume in which Zora Neale Hurston's essay "My Most Humiliating Jim Crow Experience" (1979) was published, Walker would be deeply familiar with Hurston's mistreatment by a white doctor in Brooklyn in 1931, just a decade or so before the events in "Strong Horse Tea" are set. In this short essay, Hurston describes her appointment with a white physician, who "appeared in the door all in white, looking very important, and also very unhappy from behind his round stomach" (935). Instead of being taken to an examination room, Hurston is led to a closet that houses soiled laundry, where the doctor "went through some motions, stuck a tube down my throat to extract some bile from my gall bladder, wrote a prescription and asked for twenty dollars as a fee" (936). Hurston never paid. Hurston's experience with racism at the hands of a white doctor surely would not have been lost on Walker. In fact, Walker's explanation of the strong horse tea suggests that it is a medicine of choice for those who are shut out of modern medicine. As she told an interviewer, "There's always somebody using 'strong horse tea' in the world; this day, this minute, there's some poor woman making strong horse tea for a child because she's too poor to get a doctor" (cited in Estes 221). Walker presents folk medicine not just as a vital and living tradition, but as an economic necessity. Just as Rannie is too poor to afford what is advertised in the circulars, she is too poor to get a doctor despite a "free market" of health care (Bronson and Nuridin 712).

In the mid-twentieth-century rural South, white doctors ordinarily did not "make the rounds" out to poor, rural African Americans. And there were few Black doctors practicing in the region. In the 1940s "the South had only 475 Black public health nurses, 644 Black dentists, and 2,018 Black physicians, nearly all of them in cities" (Thomas 32). In 1933, just a decade or so before the story was set, there was one physician who graduated from a medical school for every 814 people in the United States; in that same year, there were only 3805 Black physicians—one for every 3125 African Americans living in the United States (Callis 35). The number of Black physicians was even lower in the South, since many African Americans went to medical schools in the north and then stayed there after graduation. As J.A. Callis notes, writing in the *Journal of Negro Education*, "practically every large Northern city has today more colored physicians than are to be found in any one of the Southern states" (34). In 1933 in the state of Georgia, where Alice Walker was born and raised, there were 1,071,125 African Americans and only 193 Black physicians. That is one Black physician for every 5550 Black residents (Callis 35).

As Thomas has argued, legally sanctioned segregation may not have even played the principal role in the racial disparities in health; rather, it was the combination of "racism, poverty, and geographic isolation" (x), all three of which were factors for Rannie. Around the time the story was set, the death rate for African Americans from whooping cough' was approximately twice that of whites, as was the infant mortality rate (Patterson 532–533). Many white physicians practicing at this time subscribed to the belief that these health disparities pointed to an inherent inferiority in the Black body. The NAACP publication *Crises* published a conversation among six lawyers living in the South, one of whom argued that "tuberculosis and pulmonary diseases would reduce Negroes 'to inconsiderable numbers' until they eventually became extinct" (qtd. in Patterson 534). Despite the efforts of the U.S. Public Health service, the kinds of robust health departments available in large northern cities were not consistently available in the rural South until the 1950s and, as Thomas's research suggests, those that existed in the region "were typically grossly understaffed by personnel with little or no public health training, often on a part-time basis" (31).

Set against this broader historical context of widespread disparities in health access and outcomes, it is hard to interpret Walker's story as locating the blame for Snooks's death within any individual in the story—not in Rannie, who was aware of the promises of "REAL" medicine but unaware of her inability to access them; not in Sarah, whose motivations for prescribing the "horse tea" are ambiguous at best; and not even in the mailman. While he certainly bears moral culpability for his racism, even if he had delivered the message, a doctor would likely not have come. There are multiple ruptures in the systems of health, belief, and information in this story, and the remedy to a broken system is ultimately left up to the reader.

The key rupture in "Strong Horse Tea" may be the break between knowledge and action. Just like Montilla's meditation on breath, which ends by pointing to the speech that never comes, Walker's story ends with Rannie's mouth full of medicine, unaware that she'll have nobody to dispense it to. The mouth that is otherwise the vehicle of speech or breath is stopped up, and in this way, the story ends abruptly, leaving the reader to perceive the wholes from the segments and, ideally, bring the knowledge wrought by stories into action in the external world.

Conclusion

Just under 100 years separates the health crisis at the heart of Walker's text from the health crisis that Montilla and Smith document in their poem and essay, respectively. All three are primarily concerned with disruptions to breathing caused by the COVID virus, the bacterial infection that leads to whooping cough, or murder-by-suffocation, and yet all three document that a focus on the breathless body misses the larger picture. The breakdown in the respiratory system is tied up with larger breakdowns in both health and information systems. As the relentless circulation of testimonials about the miracle of ivermectin in treating COVID reminds us, the problem is not just access to information itself, but access to information *systems*. Scientific or otherwise empirical knowledge alone—about how vaccines work or about how implicit bias leads to the undertreatment of pain and unjust health outcomes for Black patients (Hoberman; The Covid Racial Data Tracker)—may treat the problem, but is not enough for a cure.

I often teach Rafael Campo's work on how poetry can help heal those living with AIDS in my Literature and Medicine class, pointing out how he is careful to distinguish the way that literature can ease the suffering of living with AIDS from an actual cure. However, as Walker, Smith, and Montilla suggest, in the case of medical racism, we may need to look outside of science for a systemic solution. Perhaps, in this case, the cure can be found in those fields that target *belief*—the humanities.

Bibliography

Bronson, Jennifer, and Tariqah Nuriddin. "'I Don't Believe in Doctors Much': The Social Control of Health Care, Mistrust, and Folk Remedies in the African American Slave Narrative." *Journal of Alternative Perspectives in the Social Sciences*, vol. 5, no. 4, 2014, pp. 706–732.

Callis, H. A. "The Need and Training of Negro Physicians." *The Journal of Negro Education*, vol. 4, no. 1, Jan. 1935, pp. 32–41.

Campo, Rafael. "Aids and the Poetry of Healing." The Kenyon Review, vol. 15, no. 4, 1993, pp. 93–100. JSTOR, http://www.jstor.org/stable/4336937. Accessed 12 November 2022.

"The Covid Racial Data Tracker." *The COVID Tracking Project*, https://covidtracking.com/race.

Estes, David C. "Alice Walker's 'Strong Horse Tea': Folk Cures for the Dispossessed." *Southern Folklore*, vol. 50, no. 3, 1 Jan. 1993, pp. 213–229.

Harley, Debra. "Indigenous Healing Practices among Rural Elderly African Americans." *International Journal of Disability, Development, and Education*, vol. 53, no. 4, December 2006, pp. 433–452.

Harris, Trudier. "Folklore in the Fiction of Alice Walker: A Perpetuation of Historical and Literary Traditions." *Black American Literature Forum*, vol. 11, no. 1, 1977, pp. 3–8.

Hoberman, John. *Black and Blue: The Origins and Consequences of Medical Racism*. U of California P, 2012.

Hooker, Deborah Anne. "Reanimating the Trope of the Talking Book in Alice Walker's 'Strong Horse Tea.'" *The Southern Literary Journal*, vol. 37, no. 2, 2005, pp. 81–102.

Hurston, Zora Neale. "My Most Humiliating Jim Crow Experience." *I Love Myself When I Am Laughing and Then Again When I Am Looking Mean & Impressive*, edited by Alice Walker, The Feminist Press at CUNY, 1979.

Martin, Dellita. "In Our Own Black Images: Afro-American Literature in the 1980s." *MELUS*, vol. 8, no. 2, Summer 1981, pp. 65–71.

Macnaughton, Jane and Havi Carel. "Breathing and Breathlessness in Clinic and Culture: Using Critical Medical Humanities to Bridge an Epistemic Gap." *The Edinburgh Companion to the Critical Medical Humanities*, edited by Anne Whitehead and Angela Woods, Edinburgh UP, 2016, pp. 294–309.

Montilla, Yesenia. "A brief meditation on breath." Poets.org, Academy of American Poets, July 21, 2020, https://poets.org/poem/brief-meditation-breath. Accessed August 16, 2022.

Patterson, Andrea. "Germs and Jim Crow: The Impact of Microbiology on Public Health Policies in Progressive Era American South." *Journal of the History of Biology*, vol. 42, no. 3, Fall 2009, pp. 529–559.

Podolsky, Scott. "The Changing Fate of Pneumonia as Public Health Concern in 20th-Century America and Beyond." *American Journal of Public Health*, vol. 95, no. 12, 2005, pp. 2144–2154.

Thomas, Karen Kruse. *Deluxe Jim Crow: Civil Rights and American Health Policy*, 1935–1954. The U of Georgia P, 2011.

Walker, Alice. "Strong Horse Tea." *Love and Trouble*, Mariner Books, 1973, pp. 88–98.

Winning, Jo. "Afterword: The Body and The Senses." *The Edinburgh Companion to the Critical Medical Humanities*, edited by Anne Whitehead and Angela Woods, Edinburgh UP, 2018, pp. 325–336.

The Mythology You Built: *After Forever*'s Narrative of Visual Desire

Lisa DeTora

Introduction

Michael Slade and Kevin Spirtas's Emmy award-winning digital series *After Forever* centers on the experiences of Brian Stone (Kevin Spirtas), a fifty-something New Yorker, after the death of his long-time partner and husband, Jason Adams (Mitchell Anderson), from stomach cancer. By depicting the loss of a legally sanctioned same-sex spouse, Slade and Spirtas also offer a new type of cultural referent that reinforces why the experiences of gay men of a certain age deserve greater cultural attention. I discuss how *After Forever* depicts Jason as an embodied being, then argue that the program creates a new way of integrating queer melancholia into a cohesive narrative of cultural and social legitimacy. *After Forever* creates a novel construction of queer melancholia that combines cultural narratives of AIDS and cancer, resituating each relative to heteronormative expectations that seek to stigmatize gay men or relegate them to

L. DeTora (✉)
Hofstra University, South Hempstead, NY, USA
e-mail: Lisa.M.DeTora@hofstra.edu

J. Cressman et al. (eds.), *Envisioning Embodiment in the Health Humanities*, Sustainable Development Goals Series,
https://doi.org/10.1007/978-3-031-49807-7_11

unhelpfully reductive homonormative or "virulent" (Dean 2007, 363) stereotypes.

Promiscuous Methodology

Theresa Geller (2013) describes "promiscuous methodological forays" (165) by foundational queer and gay critics like Alexander Doty, Eve Kosofsky Segdwick, and Robin Wood as calling into question the necessity for binary heteronormativity. Other critics like Judith Butler (2006, 2015), Sedgwick (2008), and Lauren Berlant and Michael Warner (1998) note that "garbled but powerful norms" (548) exclude certain experiences and identities without defining them, leaving a burden on queer theorists to set the terms of their own existence. However, as Sedgwick (2008) discusses, slippery definitions of sodomy *de facto* criminalized gay men, shunting their desires away from the public eye. As James Joseph Dean (2007) and Christopher Pullen (2017) observe, mainstream culture long excluded gay men, making Slade and Spirtas's goals a site of invention for which few models exist. I build on Geller's idea of promiscuous methodology to consider how various theories of looking might be brought to bear on *After Forever*, and what I see as a potentially new model of queer melancholia, which draws on prior discussions by Judith Butler (1995) and Douglas Crimp (2004).

A few major themes in looking relations are important in the current chapter. Laura Mulvey (1975) reads Hollywood films as assuming that male viewers will regard women as sexual objects. However, Caroline Evans and Lorraine Gamman (1995) called for gazes that troubled such essential gender definitions. Dean and Pullen (2017) observe that a queer gaze "coerced into the position of the voyeur" (43) creates a presence when homosexual identities were omitted or prohibited; hence, "the process of the gaze itself enables some sense of material presence" (43) for queer identities. A digital series, *After Forever* also might evoke the more domesticated and intimate televisual glance, which, as Pullen observes "offers [enhanced] scope for shared experience and interconnectivity between the audience and the text" (117). Lynne Joyrich (2014) also claims that queer television studies balance "articulation" (133) and "unsettling of the mainstream" (133). These queer gazes, then presume prohibition, which may mean that legal sanctioning of single-sex marriages might somehow shift the balance of former cultural and representational prescriptions (and proscriptions).

I suggest that *After Forever* creates a visual narrative that transforms perspectives and gazes in such a way as to create new states of understanding, being, and seeing, in part because its depictions center on a legally sanctioned single-sex marriage and in part because it assigns a gaze to a character whose states of being are both subject to change without notice and charged with framing the entire series.

In *After Forever*, what can be interpreted as Jason's gaze "after forever"—state he occupies after dying—creates a site for problematizing queer melancholia and other powerful cultural narratives and forms a new visual and cultural space for depicting married middle-aged gay men, a group that traditionally lacked straightforward access to mainstream representation. Jason's "after forever" gaze is not the only site of his perception represented in the program, making the interaction between his pre- and post-death gazes of interest. By presenting its protagonists in multiple different states of being in time and space, and using its visual and narrative representations telescope and combining lived experience, memory, and melancholia, *After Forever* creates a new representational site of gay male identity, and by extension, a new possibility for personal identity in general.

Jason as Bearer of the Look

After Forever follows a predictable, yet destabilizing, narrative structure from episode one, "Commitment," which opens on grainy video of Brian and Jason in Central Park, talking about commitment as both romantic attachment and mental illness. In the next scene, Brian and Jason awaken on their fifteenth anniversary affectionately kissing: the episode progresses from Brian's workday to an anniversary party. Brian can't imagine living without Jason, and Jason's reply "you don't have to" brings tears to all eyes. The next scene shows Brian putting one plate and a champagne flute into an empty dishwasher. And as Brian and Jason snuggle together in bed, the awful truth comes out—Jason has died. The reveal is a shock both because of the skillful visual and textual narrative construction of the episode and because of Jason's palpable physicality throughout. Each episode follows a similar pattern: Brian and Jason in Central Park (season one) or at the beach (season two), followed by an episode in Brian's life punctuated by flashbacks of his relationship with Jason and Jason's final illness (season one) or memorial service (season two).

While Jason's embodied presence could be read as grief hallucinations foreshadowed by the connection between romantic and mental health commitments, the program's visual narrative undercuts this possibility by explicitly constructing Jason's gaze at multiple points in each episode. *After Forever* creates a presence in a site of absence by rendering Jason visible and physically embodied in both life and death, and also by collapsing past and present to continually reinsert the viewer into Jason's point of view. The extent of this collapsing of time only becomes clear in the final episode of series one, "If a Man Answers" when the opening scenes in each episode in the series—Jason and Brian's first real date—are identified as what Brian describes while Jason dies in his arms. This scene collapses Brian and Jason's relationship, telescoping it into a single critical event that blends the hopeful future of new love with the devastating grief of untimely death. An astute viewer might notice that each episode not only begins with a scene that might reasonably be constructed as Jason's hazy remembrances as he passes from life but also ends from a perspective accessible exclusively to Jason's last known physical position, often watching Brian move away.

After Forever centers on Jason as an observer as much as on Brian as a protagonist. In fact, *After Forever* strongly orients the viewer to Jason's gaze, making the audience complicit in what might be seen as a type of voyeurism. For example, flashback sequences in "My Buddy," include scenes to which Brian has no access, like Jason's parting from his best friend Lisa (Cady Huffman) and quizzical looks between friends as a tear-blinded Brian staggers from Lisa's cabaret opening. The next scene shows Jason having followed Brian out into the street, which strongly suggests viewers were positioned in Jason's "after forever" point of view. Associating camera orientation and scene selection with Jason's memories or (presumed) physical location in the scene opens the possibility for the program to elide entirely the heteronormative male bearer of the look that Mulvey posited, replacing this vantage point with a gaze that wields significant social and cultural power despite the fact that Jason is only unwillingly thrust into this position. The program, then, answers earlier calls for a queer gaze that will destabilize the type of categorical gender identification inherent in Mulvey's original theory. This potential move, situating the viewer from Jason's "after forever" vantage point also may be seen as a political act, which casts Brian's experience into a nuanced cultural condition that reframes earlier narratives of queer melancholia.

Reframing Queer Melancholia

Butler (1995) described queer melancholia as the "predicament of living within a culture that can mourn the loss of homosexual attachment only with great difficulty" (166). For Butler, this difficulty lay not simply with a Freudian model of melancholia, that for her (and in contrast with Freud) informs all gendered identity formation, but with social structures that aimed to efface the possibility not only for mourning the loss of a homosexual partner, but also for having such an attachment in the first place. When homosexual partnerships are culturally proscribed, mourning for their loss is automatically "foreclosed" (165). Douglas Crimp (2004) also saw queer melancholia as impeding activism and compounded by the decimation of gay men's communities during the HIV/AIDS pandemic, a circumstance that ironically opened the possibility for mainstream media depictions of gay experience.

Sedgwick (2008) comments on the centrality of HIV/AIDS to the earliest mainstream depictions of gay men as worthy of compassion and acceptance. These men became visible only long enough to be erased, victims of what Crimp (2004) called a "magical thinking" (7) that morally sanitized gay men through tragedy, death, and/or mature acquiescence to the medical industrial complex. And this perspective is inaccessible to many today. Sedgwick notes that the "then-enveloping pressure of the AIDS emergency" (xiv) was nearly incomprehensible by the early 2000s. "It was a common experience then to be in a room of vibrant young people, conscious that within a year or two, all but a few of them would have sickened and died" (xiv-xv). Brian and Jason's community of friends are *de facto* survivors and witnesses of this critical emergency. *After Forever*, then, inverts Sedgwick's image, presenting viewers with a hopeful beginning they have no way of knowing will end in tragedy: viewers and characters enter the narrative knowing that AIDS was no longer a death sentence. *After Forever* acknowledges this past when Jason notes that his years of safe sex came to nothing ("My Buddy"), while claiming a future in which mourning the loss of a same-sex spouse has become culturally legitimated and queer points of view can reframe a powerful cultural discourse of health. The program thus telescopes not only Brian and Jason's relationship, but also their earlier experiences during the AIDS emergency.

One might think that *After Forever* sidesteps the proscription of homosexual desire and therefore avoids queer melancholia. Yet constraints on gay men's identities are still evident. "The Mouths of Babes" sees Brian and Jason discussing whether their parents accept their gayness, and David Taylor, Brian's new love interest, has parents who accept his gayness only if he is in a stable relationship ("If a Man Answers"). Tison Pugh (2017) associates these pressures to conform with stable monogamy that mimic heteronormative commitments with a desire not to alienate the sensibilities of twenty-first-century television viewers.

Many prior depictions of gay men of a certain age dovetail with a narrative that Crimp (2004) sees as the persistent adolescence of gay men. *Jeffrey*'s Sterling (Patrick Stewart), for instance, toggles between abject silliness and wanton risk-taking. In contrast, "middle-aged fag" Armand Goldman (Robin Williams) in *The Birdcage* (1996), a responsible adult, inhabits an idyllic world seemingly outside the impact of AIDS, possibly because of the film's indebtedness to its 1970s (hence, pre-HIV) French forebears. Vic Grassi (Jack Wetherall) of the US *Queer as Folk* survives to middle age only to die from complications due to his HIV medications. These representations differ strongly from Brian and Jason's circle of cultured, educated, professionally successful friends who embody a bourgeois ideal as stable, functioning members of adult society. Both Jason and Brian recognize their professional and financial privilege ("Authors"), and enact what Crimp would have seen as a foil to a model of gay identity that equated a lack of committed homonormative bonding to the sexual antics of "naughty teenaged boys" (5). The cultural equation of gayness and immaturity, thus, hints that queer melancholia resulted from an assumed failure to accept adulthood rather than a societal failure to accommodate difference.

Thus, it might seem that *After Forever* could occupy (or even create) a space located "after" the queer melancholia Butler and Crimp describe. Jason and Brian and their friends accept normative adulthood and stable monogamy yet view their marriages as political action ("Accidents," "The In-Laws"). In fact, since Brian and Jason's marriage was legally and socially recognized, and season two depicts scenes from Jason's memorial service and the scattering of his ashes, the program suggests that Brian's difficulties in mourning do not derive from a lack of legally or socially sanctioned memorializing activities. Nevertheless, Brian's predicament in negotiating a life "after forever" is evident from the first episode. While it is tempting to fall back on the idea that Brian suffers from a mental illness, like complicated grief, the program structures Brian's difficulties in two separate contexts that each reinforce the idea that *he* is not the problem. First, Jason sickened and died from cancer, a disease generally understood to follow certain medical scripts that Jason consciously rejects. Second, Brian is constructed as a site of visual pleasure, which subjects him to myriad sexual pressures and renders him into an object of sexual desire rather than a thinking subject. These narratives each resituate Brian's predicament, and Jason's, relative to melancholia, because they prevent Brian from mourning effectively.

Queering Cancer

The depiction of Jason's illness provides important clues about the problematics of melancholia in the series. Despite a diagnosis of cancer ("Back on the Bike"), Jason's experience parallels that of gay men when HIV/AIDS was incurable, the only treatment being palliative care. His physician (Collen Zenk) indicates that cure is simply not an option. Jason's stage four cancer will kill him no matter what they do. The only question is what he is willing to put himself through to gain a few extra weeks of existence. At this point, Jason's perception becomes a critical driver for narrative framing because he accepts this clinical information. This moment represents a radical break in Brian and Jason's relationship, which begins with the two men standing side by side, gazing outward together at a painting that comes to symbolize their relationship ("House for One"). The cancer diagnosis, which they also receive side by side ("Back on the Bike"), separates these long-unified gazes. The husbands' shared regard evokes Bracha Ettinger's notion of a matrixial gaze linked to the pregendered possibilities of the womb. Before cancer, Brian and Jason were linked by gazes trained on a nascent futurity and grounded in possibility.

During cancer, Jason alone bears a look that realistically accounts for medical knowledge, wielding what Foucault (1963, trans 1995) might term a clinical gaze that perceives the hitherto invisible. In Foucauldian (1963) terms, Jason hears the clinical language of diagnosis and links it to later spectacles of illness and death. In this, he reverses what Foucault described as "hearing a language" on viewing the spectacle (because the physician's language comes first). However, the linkage of language and spectacle remains important because Jason keeps himself grounded in material reality by wielding a queer gaze that fills in the future spectacles of his own death, creating a site of narcissistic voyeurism in the vein Pullen has described. Jason wields an effective clinical gaze and also this queer gaze, and it becomes evident in an argument with Brian that Jason has thought through the possible futures and chosen the least awful outcome for himself and his husband ("Back on the Bike").

In contrast, Jason's family and friends succumb to thinking that parallels the "wish fulfilment" Crimp (2004) sees in conservative interpretations of HIV/AIDS. The earlier linkage of marriage and activism again becomes important because Jason's decisions can also be seen as activism. ACT UP's *FDA Action Handbook*, as Crimp (2011), notes, focused the attention of gay men suffering from HIV/AIDS and their loved ones on medical research ethics and holding groups like the FDA accountable for following their own stated moral and professional standards. In this accounting, "healthcare is right," and *After Forever* appears to consider the question of how and when this kind of moral and ethical good should be carried out, as well as by whom.

Historically, Jason's illness falls among political currents, like Right to Try legislation, which claim that access to treatment is necessary, no matter how unlikely to succeed, or how likely to prolong or cause suffering (DeTora 2018) a sentiment seemingly echoed in comments from Jason's parents, best friend Lisa, and her husband, Andrew (Robert Emmet Lunney). Brian's initial focus on making any attempt to extend Jason's life also plays into this narrative. Jason's perception that pumping himself with "poison" in the form of chemotherapy would only deny his human dignity allows him to formulate a new narrative of cancer that resituates a necessary connection with cure espoused by characters who discuss "the chemotherapy" and "the radiation" as givens. It also allows Jason to trouble the notion that longer life is better. Instead, Jason considers *which* healthcare is right, given his circumstances. Jason's new cancer narrative, because he is a gay man faced with an incurable illness, necessarily mimics the critical emergency of AIDS he evaded as a young man, a connection he himself makes, thus reintegrating himself into a queer experience and former models of activism. At the same time, aside from a single IV stand, the program shows no medicalized visual information, which casts this medical and potentially political decision as deeply personal.

This linkage of the personal with a moral *ethos* of health as care is enacted through the rest of the series as Brian tends to his sickening and dying spouse. Significantly, other characters respect Jason's decision primarily because of Brian's unflinching support. Jason's parents only stop arguing about how Jason "can beat this" when Brian supports the decision to avoid treatment ("The In-Laws"). This acquiescence is represented as bound up in Brian's willingness to sacrifice his own feelings to his husband's quest for human dignity, even though it is clear that Brian disagrees. Brian then enacts the moral rightness of health as care, embodying Jason's vision of the best outcome in a catastrophic situation and creating what can be read as a personal site of political engagement. It is worthy of note that Brian is also the only character shown touching the IV apparatus, resituating a medical experience into his personal relationship with his dying husband. Jason's choice reinforces the necessity for dignity among gay men subject to the healthcare system while providing an unyielding look at the limits of healthcare wisdom. Furthermore, while the program clearly highlights Jason's bravery in the face of his final illness and premature death, it is unclear whether any of the other characters appreciate his actions, because the indicators of his emotions are presented outside their lines of sight.

Jason's reframing of the cancer narrative also squarely situates Brian in a site of queer melancholic experience that these characters thought they had avoided. Brian's experience, however, unlike that Crimp (2004) describes, causes the death only of his most cherished personal connection, which then creates a novel site of melancholia. The AIDS emergency devastated whole communities—Crimp notes that not only his inner circle but even the professional and social peripheries of his life were decimated. In contrast, Brian's experience is individual, which creates considerable pressure to move on after his bereavement ("Accidents," "My Buddy"). In fact, Brian's struggle may have more to do with an inability to discuss his suppressed anger, an emotion evident from the initial episode, than a lack of sanctioned mourning opportunities, a circumstance that finds a parallel in Butler's observation that queer melancholia also forecloses the possibility for anger.

If, as Butler notes, "the rage over the loss can redouble by being unavowed" (178), then Brian's predicament is serious not only because he quite clearly is angry but also because, by embodying and supporting Jason's decision, he subsumed his own opinion, presenting an outward appearance of agreement. And this personal collapse into another signals an important struggle for Brian: when lesbian work wife Brenda (Erin Cherry) criticizes his apparent adoption of Italian widowhood, clinging not only to Jason's memory but also to his underpants ("Accidents"), Brian notes that he and Jason didn't have separate underwear. Thus, when Brian says "Fuck you. No, fuck ***cancer***" to Jason's picture, even Brenda fails to honor this initial impulse in part because Brian's identity is so entirely tied up with Jason's. Ironically, Jason's best friend Lisa blames

Brian for not insisting that Jason get treatment, leaving Brian not only unable to express his own anger but also having to manage hers ("My Buddy"). Thus, Brian's ability to express anger is foreclosed not by a proscription against his marriage, but by the fact that his marriage superposed his identity with Jason's, creating not "his" but "our" life, and leaving his personal preferences visible only to Jason ("Back on the Bike").

Ultimately, Brian's post bereavement narrative is constrained not just by accepted healthcare narratives but also by the reality that he, like Jason, may only choose a best quality of life, not a cure. Borrowing again from Foucault, Jason's medical gaze creates a situation that transforms Brian and Jason's marriage into a new state of being that at first reduces Brian to an embodiment of health care delivery and later transforms Jason to an unwilling voyeur and casts Brian adrift as an object of desire rather than a mutually desiring subject. Brian is unable to reclaim a single life because he remains bound to Jason, responsible for the emotional management of Jason's other significant attachments, including his parents ("The In-Laws"), best friend Lisa, and even Jason's protegee and former lover, Stefan, who seeks Brian's professional help ("Authors"). Brian's ongoing responsibility for Jason's legacy forestalls discussions about keeping reasonable boundaries between his dead husband's long-ago sexual infidelity and the workplace, an echo of earlier comments about Brian wearing Jason's clothes ("Accidents") as well as future observations that engaging in a sexual relationship with Brian is tantamount to a "threeway" ("Goodbyes").

Brian, then, is unwillingly thrust into an unstable terrain of dating while in an undefined state himself, enjoined to decide what he "really wants" when that desire, his husband, will never be available. And Brian finds that dating balances questions of open relationships, monogamy, partnerships, boyfriends, friends who have sex, fuck buddies, and marriage as necessarily negotiated and overlapping, a situation further complicated by the idea that remarrying after a spouse's death might constitute bigamy ("Define Cheating"). In other words, Brian must find a way to construct a viable relationship, including its model of desire, while he is reconstructing a personal identity that must still carry out obligations incurred during his marriage and that keep him bound up in his shared identity with Jason. This situation, then, places him in a new relationship to a queer melancholia that is fueled in part by the very institutions whose exclusion of gay men framed the condition originally described by Crimp and Butler.

Brian as Object of Desire

The second problem Brian must face is a desire for a stable union. An ongoing critique of certain cultural constructions is that they insert stereotypical same-sex pairings into otherwise heteronormative forms and thereby subsume the transgressive and transformative potential of queer culture into the troublesome binaries that necessitated the formation of antiheteronormative counterknowledge in the first place. The opening of *After Forever* suggests that Brian, Jason and their friends inhabit such conservative "good gay" models. However, their dialogue reveals more nuanced understandings. In "Commitment," Peter (Peter Y. Kim) and Mark (Jonathan Rayson), Brian and Jason's married neighbors, trouble the notion of "breeder" as a solely heteronormative domain, which is a site for a possibility Pugh sees when "conservatism is not the monolithically patriarchal force that it once was" (24). Yet Mark and Peter's gambit hints at a challenging terrain of personal identity formation that Brian must navigate after losing a stable marriage. The queer terrain that Brian enters does not present this "good gay" model as an automatic option.

As a widower, Brian is faced with sexual liaisons that will never come close to filling the void created by Jason's death because of a persistent cultural identification of gay sex as the behavior of naughty adolescents. In "Commitment," for example, Brian's masseuse jerks him off, an encounter that obtrudes like a trauma in "My Buddy," when Brian's friend Paul (Jamison Stern) recommends Grindr as a sexual outlet. Paul, a former sex buddy of Brian's, has a great deal of difficulty not discussing his memories of Brian's penis in public despite their lack of sexual contact in more than fifteen years. This slippage hints at consistent outside pressure and competition within Brian's friend group that placed pressures on his marriage that extend beyond Jason's death. For example, Lisa competes with Brian for Jason's emotional intimacy, even after Jason has died. Paul's ongoing fascination, at least discursively, with Brian's genitalia, also signals further tensions that play out in attempts to fix Brian up with romantic partners in the face of an early sexual fiasco.

Whereas, as Crimp (2004) writes, earlier moments in gay men's history sexually marginalized middle-aged men, Brian is subject to near-constant sexual attention. Younger colleagues compliment Brian flirtatiously, and the receptionist "mistakenly" sends Brian's mail to a young man who is clearly attracted to him. Waiters in Paul's restaurant also express interest, as does Ron (Jim Newman), a casual passer-by during a Saturday bike ride, who later approaches Brian on the street outside his workplace and initiates a sexual relationship. When Ron's committed open relationship to another man is revealed in front of Brian's friends (and Ron's partner of three years), a cascade of fix ups ensues. The possibilities range from twenty-something waiters chosen by friend Paul (who asks for details) to age-appropriate realtors offered by Peter and Mark. In the face of Brenda's matter-of-fact assertion that lots of people have open relationships, however, Brian quietly discards the phone numbers. This behavior has parallels in his early relationship with Jason, who, clearly attracted to Brian, approaches him, and initiates physical contact, then asks him out for a drink. Season one ends with Brian's first date with David (Mike McGowan), the handsome son of friends of Jason's parents, who calls only after confirming Brian's attractiveness on social media. Although Jason's gaze is not the only means of rendering Brian into an object of sexual desire, the primacy of this relationship is evident when Brian, having just met the handsome, charming David, poignantly exchanges a look with a clearly upset Jason. This scene calls on Jason to put aside his feelings in the service of the man he loves, linking them together in a cycle of mutual self-sacrifice.

Yet, while Brian will always be Jason's "forever," Brian must make a decision about whether or not Jason will be his. By season two, David has become Brian's romantic "something" and begins to integrate Brian into a new world of intersectional possibilities. Viewers learn that David, an architect, is the seemingly "good gay" outlier in a community of queer thinkers who reject the age-matched normativity Brian and Jason's friend group exhibit, actively questioning the emotional and sexual logic of permanent monogamous coupling ("Honeymoon"). David's friends enact romantic relationship models that Brian had explicitly rejected. While Lisa and her husband Andrew laughingly trouble their heteronormative standing by rejecting not the "hetero" but the "norm," Peter and Mark calmly integrate themselves within these conversations, seamlessly situating Mark's job as a schoolteacher relative to that of David's friend, Clifford (Michael McElroy), who teaches African American literature at Columbia, and who met his partner of three years, a twenty-something recent college graduate, in class. Another problem for Brian in negotiating these new possibilities is where and how he can include a new partner in his life, as Jason's physical presence becomes increasingly more problematic.

In season one, Jason's palpable presence seemed not unwelcome during tax audits, breakfast, bicycling with a friend, waking up or going to sleep, but in season two having sex and building a connection with a new partner seem to call for an added measure of privacy. The viewer, like Brian and David's friends, are invited into the relationship only in the opening of season two ("Honeymoon"), which begins six months after the couple's first date. The day their friends are supposed to meet, Jason interferes with Brian's shaving routine while David showers, leaving Brian to balance two conversations, a situation that becomes more chaotic when Jason begins to enter the bedroom while David and Brian make love. The season two opener also sees David occupying Jason's place in Brian's bed and closes with Jason, seated at the kitchen counter, watching Brian lead David to their bedroom. This spot at the counter is later shown to be where Brian was sitting when he first accused Jason of having an affair with Stefan, and where Jason was standing when he confessed the affair ("Authors"). By the time David, sitting by the kitchen counter in the exact spot Brian occupied to confront Jason about his infidelity, comments that he feels like he is in "a threeway" ("Goodbyes"), the new relationship is on the rocks. David clearly does not want to part from Brian, but Brian is not ready to move on. It is Jason, who, crouching in the bedroom while David occupies his space in Brian's bed, reveals the unwelcome truth that the "mythology" Brian built up about their marriage has become exaggerated, leaving Brian not only without Jason, but also without accurate memories of their relationship.

It also becomes clear that although Jason encourages Brian to move on, he is simultaneously unwilling to leave Brian's presence. As Brian begins to box up the myriad mementos and images of their marriage, his eye falls on the painting that brought them together in the first place, then further cemented their bond as an anniversary gift ("House for One"). This moment also signals a further significant shift when the sight of the painting triggers Brian's romantic perception, showing him that "David is right." Once again, the possibility opens for a new, mutual relationship where two clear-sighted partners can face outward together, as Jason and Brian did from their first meeting until Jason's death—even in the face of Jason's infidelity ("Authors"). David's observations offer Brian new access to romantic perception, an ability to see what is before him and not to dwell only on what is absent. Jason's interference, at first verbal, becomes physical; however, his words "I'll take care of you," forestall any further connection because they form another site of collapse, linking visually and thematically with the moment when Jason refuses cancer treatment ("Back on the Bike") and Brian relinquishes his own judgment in the service of his marriage. Jason is positioned in the exact spot where he stood when refusing treatment, despite Brian's pleas. The present-day narrative ends with Brian's angry look at his now-dead husband.

The series then segues to its final scene, when Brian scatters Jason's ashes at the site of their honeymoon trip. As Brian releases his husband's remains, and himself, Jason's embodied presence appears, and Brian's bewildered, teary expression is flabbergasted, not welcoming. This moment, like Jason's death, telescopes the most joyful and painful moments of their relationship, collapsing pleasure and pain, while reinforcing the power of Jason's presence and his gaze to influence Brian's life. It also, belatedly, informs the viewer that the opening of the series is set quite recently after Jason's reappearance. In effect, Brian was repositioned from freedom to a permanent state of melancholia in the light of that impish gaze. This final moment simultaneously reflects Brian's irresistible pull (in the preceding episode Ron leaves his long-term lover to pursue Brian) as well as his perplexity at becoming an object of desire rather than an equal partner. Significantly, both moments construct Brian as the object of Jason's gaze, keeping the viewer situated in a site of his unwilling voyeurism, revealing nothing of Brian's thoughts and leaving the future uncertain.

Conclusion

After Forever presents several constructions of queer melancholia that I figured through a methodologically promiscuous theorizing of a gaze that relies on a subtle insertion of the viewer into Jason's unwilling voyeurism. This positioning allows the series to present a model of Jason and Brian's love relationship that telescopes courtship, marriage, death and memorial, transforming each of these activities into a model of mourning that, while legally and culturally sanctioned, might remain a site of permanent melancholic associations. Yet this interpretation belies a more cheerful narrative, which is that by resituating moments of death and memorial in terms of the promise of new connection, the series also opens the possibility for Brian to release Jason and take up a new partnership. The intersectionality of Brian's expanded friend group also presents further sites for new, constructive experiences that are not constrained by "good gay" expectations modelled in heteronormative coupling. Further transformations are evident in Jason's reframing of a cancer narrative that can be seen to restore a site of queer activism in medicine as well as Brian's enactment of an ethics of health care as morally right. Each of these affordances relies on the visual and narrative construction of Jason's gaze as a frame for the program and as a consumer of healthcare information. Ultimately, the series illustrates that while not all situations result in happy outcomes, hope and human dignity may support choices that reaffirm the quality of life no matter what the situation.

Bibliography

Berlant, Lauren, and Michael Warner, "Sex in Public,." *Critical Inquiry*, vol. 24, no. 2, 1998, pp. 547–566.

Butler, Judith. *Bodies That Matter: On the Discursive Limits of Sex*. Routledge, 2015.

Butler, Judith. *Gender Trouble: Feminism and the Subversion of Identity*. Routledge, 2006.

Butler, Judith. "Melancholy Gender-Refused Identification." *Psychoanalytic Dialogues*, vol. 5, no. 2, 1995, pp. 165–180.

Crimp, Douglas. *Melancholia and Moralism*. MIT Press, 2004.

Crimp, Douglas. "Before Occupy: How AIDS Activists Seized Control of the FDA in 1988" The Atlantic. Dec 6, 2011. https://www.theatlantic.com/health/archive/2011/12/before-occupy-how-aids-activists-seized-control-of-the-fda-in-1988/249302/

Dean, James Joseph. "Gays and Queers: From the Centering to the Decentering of Homosexuality in American Films." *Sexualities*, vol. 10, no. 3, 2007, pp. 363–386. https://doi.org/10.1177/1363460707078337.

DeTora, Lisa. "The Dangers of Magical Thinking: Situating Right to Try Laws, Patient's Rights, and the Language of Advocacy." *Rhetoric of Health and Medicine*, vol. 1, nos. 1–2, 2018, pp. 37–57.

Evans, Caroline and Lorraine Gamman. "The Gaze Revisited, or Reviewing Queer Viewing." *A Queer Romance: Lesbians, Gay Men and Popular Culture*, edited by Paul Burston and Colin Richardson, Routledge, 1995.

Foucault, Michel. (1963). *The Birth of the Clinic: An Archaeology of Medical Perception*, translated by A. M. Sheridan Smith. Vintage, 1995.

Geller, Teresa L. "Is Film Theory Queer Theory? Or, Everything I Know about Queerness I Learned at the Movies." *Camera Obscura: Feminism, Culture, and Media Studies*, vol. 28, no. 3, 2013, pp. 159–167.

Joyrich, Lynn, "Queer Television Studies: Currents, Flows, and (Main) streams."*Cinema Journal*, vol. 53, no. 2, 2014, pp. 133–139.

Mulvey, Laura. "Visual Pleasure and Narrative Cinema." *Screen*, vol. 16, no. 4, 1975, pp. 6–18.

Pugh, Tison (2017). "Conservative Narrativity, Queer Politics, and the Humor of Gay Stereotypes in Modern Family", Camera Obscura, vol. 32, no. 3, pp. 1–31, https://doi.org/10.1215/02705346

Pullen, Christopher. *Straight Girls and Queer Guys: The Hetero Media Gaze in Film and Television*. Edinburgh UP, 2017.
Sedgwick, Eve K. *Epistemology of the Closet*. U of California P, 2008.
Slade, Michael. "Accidents" *After Forever*, Season 1, Episode 4.
Slade, Michael. "Authors" *After Forever*, Season 2, Episode 7.
Slade, Michael. "Back on the Bike" *After Forever*, Season 1, Episode 2.
Slade, Michael. "Commitment" *After Forever*, Season 1, Episode 1.
Slade, Michael. "Define Cheating" *After Forever*, Season 1, Episode 6.
Slade, Michael. "Goodbyes" *After Forever*, Season 2, Episode 8.
Slade, Michael. "Honeymoon" *After Forever*, Season 2, Episode 1.
Slade, Michael. "If a Man Answers" *After Forever*, Season 1, Episode 8.
Slade, Michael. "My Buddy" *After Forever*, Season 1, Episode 3.
Slade, Michael. "The In-Laws" *After Forever*, Season 1, Episode 7.
(2017) Conservative Narrativity Queer Politics and the Humor of Gay Stereotypes in Modern Family Camera Obscura: Feminism Culture and Media Studies 32(3) 1-31 10.1215/02705346-4205055

Dead Matter: COVID-19 and the Banning of Burials in Sri Lanka

Shalini Abayasekara

Introduction

On December 9, 2020, Sri Lanka's youngest Coronavirus victim up to that point, twenty-day-old Shaykh, was cremated against his parents' will. Shaykh's parents had Shaykh after a six-year wait. Some days later, however, they noticed that the baby was struggling to breathe, and rushed him to hospital. They were first told their baby was suffering from pneumonia, but later, were told that he was COVID-positive. Despite the parents' tears and pleas for more detailed examination they were sent home. The

I myself am not Muslim but am part of Sri Lanka's Christian minority. Thus, I do not write from personal experience as a Muslim, but from my observations and experiences having lived and grown up in Sri Lanka, often in multicultural settings. Arguably, someone from a different positionality would have somewhat different reflections on the "situation."

S. Abayasekara (✉)
The Ohio State University, Columbus, OH, USA
e-mail: abayasekara.1@buckeyemail.osu.edu

J. Cressman et al. (eds.), *Envisioning Embodiment in the Health Humanities*, Sustainable Development Goals Series,
https://doi.org/10.1007/978-3-031-49807-7_12

next day, they were informed that Shaykh had died of the illness. Shaykh's father Mohamed Fahim repeatedly asked the doctors to conduct a PCR test to reconfirm this, but to no avail. He was not handed back his child's body either. Instead, he was asked to sign a document authorizing Shaykh's cremation (which he refused to do). The following day, he was informed that Shaykh's body was being taken to the crematorium ("COVID-19: Sri Lanka" 2020).

This enforced cremation resulted from a "burial ban" Sri Lanka's government implemented during the COVID-19 pandemic, a ban that gravely affected Sri Lanka's Muslim community, to which Shaykh and his family belonged.[1] Before examining the ban's history and implications, however, I will define some key concepts and theories I employ in this chapter. One such concept is embodiment. Embodiment has sometimes been equated with corporeality—"the state of living in/through/as a body" (Wilkerson 2015, 67). Tanya Titchkosky (2020), writing from a disability studies perspective, defines embodiment as a complex web of relations that one develops by having and being bodies, which connects to how meanings become associated with people. Jay Timothy Dolmage explores the intersections of disability and rhetoric, and argues that embodiment is "always a mode of persuasion" if one notes that all meaning comes from the body, and that communication in turn shapes the body's possibilities (2014, 89). Body and mind are thus interconnected, a linkage particularly apparent in the term "bodymind" (Price).

In short, then, embodiment involves how "people (acting in their bodies) relate and assign meaning to other people and bodies" (Swacha 2018, 261). Considering these ways of understanding embodiment, this chapter regards embodiment in terms of how bodies (or "bodyminds") engage with other bodies/bodyminds to make meaning. I examine the complexity of relations involved in having and being bodies, and the ways those complex relations between different bodies play out in a crisis like a pandemic.

[1] In terms of religion, Sri Lanka comprises Buddhists (70.2%), Hindus (12.6%), Muslims (9.7%), and Christians (7.4%) (US Department of State, Office of International Religious Freedom). Buddhists belong to the Sinhala ethnic group (thereby making the "Sinhala Buddhist" ethnoreligious category the largest in the country), Hindus to the Tamil ethnic group, Muslims to the Islam/Moor group, and Christians to either the Sinhala, Tamil, or Burgher group (i.e., there are Sinhala Christians, Tamil Christians, and a small minority of Burgher Christians). The country's population is currently estimated at roughly 21.5 million.

The "rhetorical situation" offers a useful framework to consider how meanings were attributed in Sri Lanka during COVID-19 to certain bodies, and how those meanings affected (or likely affected) these individuals thus embodied. The concept "rhetorical situation" refers to "any set of circumstances that involves at least one person using some sort of communication to modify the perspective of at least one other person" ("Rhetorical Situations" 2022). Thus as Lloyd Bitzer (1968), one of the earliest theorists on the rhetorical situation, notes, a rhetorical situation cannot exist unless its circumstances (or "exigences"—urgent needs/demands) can be modified using language. Exigences like seasonal changes or natural disasters, the existence of which language cannot change, do not constitute a rhetorical situation.

Turning to theories about the rhetorical situation, Bitzer sees the rhetorical situation as giving rise to discourse. He argues for the existence of a situation apart from any human interpretation of it via language, stating that if there is discourse, there must obviously be a situation that requires the discourse. Richard Vatz, on the other hand, approaches the rhetorical situation as myth. He argues that statements about situations do not indicate the situation's characteristics, but "only inform us as to the phenomenological perspective of the speaker" (1973, 154). For him, there is no situation with a nature independent of the *speaker's* view or the *speaker*'s language used to characterize it.

Barbara Biesecker moves the focus away from the debate regarding the situation versus rhetor as creating meaning. Part of her focus is audience, and she states that the rhetorical event may be considered as producing and reproducing identities of, and linkages between, audience members. There is no predetermined audience body with a fixed identity, simply induced to act one way or another. Instead, the rhetorical situation enables "the production of identities and social relations" (1989, 126). Jenny Edbauer's (2005) work on the rhetorical situation takes these theorizations even further. Edbauer uses the term "rhetorical ecologies," explaining that the rhetorical situation is better conceptualized as a mixture of processes and encounters, involving many different occurrences that are not properly segmented into audience, text, and rhetorician. There is emphasis on the various factors at play within this ecology, and these factors' relationship to time and history.

In this chapter, I explore how theories about the rhetorical situation help understand the burial ban and the resultant embodiment of Sri Lanka's Muslim population. Specifically, I examine how, by prohibiting the burial of COVID-19 victims, the ban framed Sri Lanka's Muslim population—for whom burial is crucial—as potentially non-compliant and dangerous. Some questions I explore are: What meanings are attributed through the ban's enactment to the Muslim body? How do theories about the rhetorical situation help understand this attribution of meaning? What role do stigma and discrimination play in this attribution?

The Burial Ban

Returning to the enforced cremation of baby Shaykh, one might say that Shaykh was born at the wrong time in the wrong place. In March 2020, with the increasing spread of the Coronavirus, the Sri Lankan government introduced a ban on burying the bodies of those who had died due to COVID-19. The reason given was that burials could contaminate underground water and thus exacerbate the virus' spread. Shreen Saroor (2020) and Dawood et al. (2020) note that a circular published on March 27 allowed for cremation or burial within twenty four hours; however, the Ministry of Health's *Provisional Clinical Practice Guidelines on COVID-19 Suspected and Confirmed Patients*, dated March 31, made cremation the only option. These provisional guidelines were then reinforced on April 11 by a further regulation in legal terms, regarding the mandatory nature of cremation.

The ban, as mentioned, gravely affected one minority group in Sri Lanka—the Muslim community. While the country's Christian minority also often bury their dead, for Muslims doing so is crucial. Cremation is deemed a form of mutilation, forbidden by Allah. Moreover, cremation is seen as sacrilegious not just for the dead individual but for the entire community of believers. Al-Dawoody and Finegan (2020) note that burying the dead is a collective obligation (*farḍ kifāyah*) in Islam. Therefore, besides the grief and despair caused by the combination of a loved one's death, such death during a pandemic, and the inability to follow core deathcare practices (Dawood et al. 2020), this collective responsibility for burial meant that the entire Muslim community would be guilty if this duty went unfulfilled.

Due to these beliefs about burial, the ban also likely discouraged Muslims from seeking treatment, out of fear about forced cremation should they die of the disease (Shaheed et al. 2021; Slater and Fonseka 2021; "Small fear" 2020; "Sri Lanka finally lifts ban on burial of COVID victims" 2021; "Sri Lanka's cremation" 2021). Statistics show that this discouragement indeed seems to have been the case. Published eleven months after the ban, Al-Jazeera's news article "Sri Lanka finally lifts ban on burial of COVID victims" reports that according to Muslim community leaders, more than half the country's 459 COVID-19 victims at the time were from the Muslim minority—a disproportionate number considering that Muslims make up just 9.7% of the country's population. Even in the early stages of the pandemic, Muslim victims were reported as comprising almost half of the country's full Coronavirus death toll ("Small fear").

In fact, the Muslim community seems to have been specifically targeted by the ban. Saroor and Dawood et al. point out that while, until March 30, the Ministry of Health webpage listed burial as a safe option for COVID-19 victims, the guidelines changed on March 31, following the death of the first Muslim victim (who was subjected to a rushed cremation without their loved ones' consent). Though Muslim leaders requested that the prime minister appoint a committee of experts to investigate the possibility of burial, even one and a half months later, nothing had been done. Similarly, Director-General of Health Dr. Jasinghe ignored a request that he consult a team of experts regarding the absence of proof that burial constituted a public health hazard. The request was made by the largest body that represents government doctors—the Government Medical Officers Association. Statements from the College of Community Physicians of Sri Lanka, the Sri Lanka Medical Association, and world-renowned virologist (and Sri Lankan) Prof. Malik Peiris (Shaheed et al.; "Covid-19: Sri Lanka" 2021) were also disregarded.

Several international organizations then argued that the ban constituted a human rights violation. A report by the University of Minnesota Law School Human Rights Clinic (UMLSHRC 2021) stated that Sri Lanka's Supreme Court did not consider constitutional and religious freedom arguments and dismissed evidence of the practices of 189 countries permitting burial, the findings of the World Health Organization, and scientific studies concluding that burial could be safely implemented. United Nations human rights experts, later also quoted by Amnesty International, called the ban a decision "based on discrimination, aggressive nationalism and ethnocentrism amounting to persecution of Muslims and other minorities in the country" (Amnesty International 2021, 5; Shaheed et al.). Many sources (Amnesty International [2021]; Ethirajan [2019]; Saroor [2020]; "Small fear" [2020]; "Sri Lanka's cremation" [2021]; Srinivasan [2020]; UMLSHRC [2021]) also linked the ban to a long-standing pattern of discrimination against Muslims by the government and/or Sinhala Buddhist extremist groups, involving the community's criminalization and even demonization.

Notably, early global guidelines regarding COVID-19 do mention dangers of water contamination through burial. For example, an article by Finegan et al. as part of the International Committee of the Red Cross states that "burial in single graves is the preferred method of disposal [as opposed to cremating unidentified human remains], but care must be taken to ensure that run-off from the decomposing human remains is managed so as not to contaminate groundwater" (2020, 132). However, nowhere is safely implemented burial prohibited (and as Dawood et al. note, there are times when burial over cremation is *recommended*, for example to minimize air pollution). Finegan et al. also emphasize the need to consult with relevant stakeholders, especially religious representatives, to ensure that changes to general deathcare practices are acceptable. And in fact, while legislation around enforced cremation was introduced in the United Kingdom as well, it was soon amended, on March 23, 2020, with the realization of how it would affect the country's Jewish and Muslim communities ("Coronavirus: UK amends emergency bill" 2020). The Sri Lankan government, however, introduced the ban a week later.

Scapegoating and Othering

Not only were Sri Lanka's Muslims discriminated against by the ban, but they were also sometimes made scapegoats for the virus' presence and diffusion. In May 2020 Saroor writes that "two private media channels currently appear hell-bent on branding Muslims as the introducers, carriers and spreaders of COVID-19 in Sri Lanka." Similarly, UMLSHRC notes that the pandemic gave rise to misinformation spread by social media and by government actors, including false allegations that Muslim businesses were intentionally spreading the disease. The UMLSHRC also cites the Alliance of Independent Professionals, a group of Sri Lankan academics and professionals, who highlighted the stigmatization resulting from certain quarantined groups being labeled as those from Muslim-predominant areas. For example, the town Beruwela in the Kalutara district is closely associated with Muslims because Beruwela is the location of the country's first Muslim settlement. And those quarantined due to COVID in the Kalutara district were labeled "Beruwela people," signaling a conflation of race and disease (aptly described by the term "name-blaming" David Craig [2020] uses when discussing naming in the 1918 "Spanish flu"). Also according to UMLSHRC, TV presenter Chatura Alwis mentioned that two Coronavirus patients from Beruwala had "deprived Sri Lanka of enjoying Sinhala New Year" (2021, 5).[2] UMLSHRC highlights a statement by the Ministry of Health's consultant pathologist as well, that the mandatory cremation policy was sparked by a fear that dead bodies would be used as biological weapons. Though not an accusation explicitly aimed at any single group, the statement arguably targeted a community that does not cremate its dead—such as Muslims.

Such scapegoating and Othering—the view of a group as intrinsically different from and alien to oneself—did not occur only in Sri Lanka during the pandemic. Slater and Masih describe the assault on a harmless Muslim man in New Delhi, reports of discrimination and attacks on people of Asian origin in the United States and Europe, and evictions of Africans in China, due to apparent fears of Coronavirus infection. Even within the Muslim community discrimination occurred; for instance, activists note that in Pakistan the Hazara ethnic minority was blamed as the virus' source (Slater and Masih 2020).

Othering during a large scale disease is not new either. In her now-classic study *AIDS and Its Metaphors*, Susan Sontag discusses how the metaphors used to describe AIDS, specifically militaristic metaphors like "war" and "defend," work to Other minoritized communities and thereby justify state-sponsored repression and violence. Sontag notes that such metaphors "implement the way particularly dreaded diseases are envisaged as an alien "other"…and the move from the demonization of the illness to the attribution of fault to the patient is an inevitable one, no matter if the patients are thought of as victims" (1989, 11). Diseases are attributed "meaning"—as, for instance, representing a curse or punishment. The different becomes the wrong.

This Othering also means that the "general population" often does not concern itself with a disease unless the disease is in its immediate vicinity. Sontag remarks that AIDS "quickly became a global event" because it became associated with "famous countries" (1989, 83). If not for this, it would have been seen as part of the "natural cycle" African and Asian countries regrettably experience, for which nothing can really be done by more resource-rich countries (1989, 83–84). This observation, made over three decades previously, is striking in its similarity to Marius Meinhof's argument in his 2020 article "Othering the Virus." In this article Meinhof

[2] The Sinhala and Tamil New Year is a celebration that takes place in April among the country's Sinhala and Tamil communities (though Tamil is excluded from Alwis' comment here, as is often—very problematically—the case).

highlights the lackadaisical approach to the news of the Coronavirus European nations took. He notes that initially, these nations deemed the virus simply a phenomenon affecting the Chinese Other and one that, even if appearing in Europe, would not be as great a calamity to *Europeans* given their superior resources. Meinhof remarks that "[d]espite the fears of some 'China-Experts', 'we' did not see a great threat, because 'we' perceived the virus as something related to the Chinese authoritarian or backward other, disconnected from the West."

Foregrounding such discriminatory Othering and scapegoating within conceptualizations of the rhetorical situation, I will now examine how Sri Lanka's burial ban framed Muslims as potentially non-compliant and therefore dangerous. Embodiment is especially useful for approaching this framing as it helps one contemplate how the ban led to various meanings made of the Muslim body and the reactions, thereby, incurred towards Muslims by other bodies. What meanings does the ban's enactment attribute to the Muslim body? How do theories about the rhetorical situation help understand this attribution of meaning? What role does stigma and discrimination play in this attribution?

The Rhetorical Situation Applied

As described before, the Bitzerian view of the rhetorical situation takes an event as given—as existing objectively. Therefore, if one were to examine the ban and the resultant embodiment of the Muslim community through this lens, one could say the Sri Lankan government genuinely believed that the pandemic necessitated cremation. The "objectively identifiable" situation was that burial could contaminate underground water and thereby increase the virus' spread. According to this understanding, then, one would not say any "special" meaning was associated with the Muslim body. One simply had to follow the rules in a time of crisis, Muslim or not.

Indeed, some of these views were expressed in comments to a news article published even before the ban was made official. In this article, the writer Haaris Mahmud (2020) pleads with the president to refrain from enacting the plan of enforced cremation, detailing faith-based reasons for his request. But some responses to this article term this plea as displaying a "really selfish, anti-national attitude." Muslims are told that they "can't expect themselves to be above everyone else, bloody hell!" and that they need to "learn to respect society or get the hell out" (Ronnie 2020). Another comment, albeit considerably less intense, reads "In ordinary times, people can practice their ordinary cultural and religions [sic] practices. In extraordinary times, people need to follow extraordinary measures to save themselves" (Amarasiri 2020). There is also outright sarcasm alongside disbelief that burial poses no extraordinary risk: "'Burning of dead body [sic] is considered a form of mutilation by Allah'. But circumcision is not considered a form of mutilation by Allah. What a hypocrisy" (Lanka Perera 2020).

But if one examines the ban through a Vatzian perspective, the objectivity of the situation that burial *was* dangerous becomes questionable. This situation of unsafety seems rather to have been *created* by the government through quoting supposed—but unverified—risks in burial. Moreover, and importantly, while Vatz's theory conceptualizes instances where the rhetor believes their interpretation to be accurate, in the case of the ban, the existence of such genuine belief is doubtful. Instead, as highlighted in both local and international media, the ban seemed to many a purposeful act of discrimination towards Muslims by the Sri Lankan government.

Lerita Coleman Brown's application of Erving Goffman's key concept "stigma" offers a useful perspective through which to view such discrimination and the resultant shaping of Othered bodies. Coleman Brown writes that "[s]tigma represents a view of life; a set of personal and social constructs; a set of social relations and social relationships; a form of social reality" (2013, 147). By forbidding burial, the government criminalized burial and constructed those who resisted the regulation as not just different but criminal. The ban capitalized on "devalued, feared" differences (Coleman Brown 147), fueling the racialization of Muslims and categorizing the Muslim body as Other, including the Other in terms of beliefs and rituals.[3] Bodies were coded (e.g., as threatening) in ways that served political interests so that, as Cressman and DeTora (2021) note can occur, injustice was "naturalized." The ban also insidiously *merged* types of fear towards difference; some likely did not even realize that underlying concerns of the Muslim minority "taking over" the country—a subtly disseminated but well-known narrative in Sri Lanka—were utilized to create scientifically baseless worries of the virus' spread.

[3] See the insightful discussion in the article "The imperative for examining anti-Muslim racism in rhetorical studies" by Yousuf and Calafell (2018) for an explanation of how Muslims can be regarded as a racialized group, existing at the intersections of a religious identity and racial identity and undergoing structural inequality and violence.

Despite such meanings potentially attributed to Muslims through the ban, the audiences, as Biesecker would say, were not entirely passive or pre-determined. If one were to believe the ban had a discriminatory agenda, then it seems as though the government did subscribe a certain pre-existing Muslim identity to those of Muslim faith and sought to do something that would violate the community's beliefs (and thus its identity). Yet one could also argue that the ban *created* or *strengthened* a particular Muslim identity—an identity protesting the ban, unified as a collective. Furthermore, the ban's condemnation by Muslims internationally (e.g., Al-Dawoody; Marsoof [2022]; Shaheed [2021]; Siddiqui and Nozell [2021]) indicates that this collective body, and its retaliations to the situation's "speaker," were not limited to local Muslims.

The ban's audiences were also not just Muslims. There were, for instance, those from other ethno-religious groups who condoned and even supported the ban. "Covid-19: Sri Lanka" discusses the ban as fulfilling the racist agenda of a few, while the comments to Mahmud's article, some of which were noted above, indicate agreement with this agenda or genuine concern over burial's apparent risk. These collectives did not exist prior to the ban, at least as a group against Muslim burial practices, but were formed by the ban into a body. Both groups, one could say—the believing and the non-believing but manipulating—were likely the government's vague "target audiences." But once baby Shaykh's case occurred, many previously unsympathetic or indifferent individuals united in the *opposite* direction ("Covid 19: Sri Lanka"; Srinivasan). They protested the government's ban rather than agreeing with the given reason of unsafe burials, tying white cloths symbolically on cemetery gates. There were also those who had rejected the ban all along. Thus, we could even think of "*anti*-audiences" in relation to the ban's supposed rationale: a collective body against Othering and discrimination.

The instigation of these anti-audiences through baby Shaykh's cremation highlights the potential significance of a baby's body. "Covid-19: Sri Lanka" (2020) quotes Amnesty International researcher Thyagi Ruwanpathirana, who was among those tying white cloths on the cemetery gates after Shaykh's cremation. In a tweet about her experience, Ruwanpathirana stated: "While I was tying it, a mother and daughter duo crossed the road and joined me with their own white cloths. Till I came they were worried someone may be watching. I couldn't quite make out what the mother was trying to say at first…Then she said, 'The baby was only two-days-old no?[4] Sin.[5] This way at least my heart will be satisfied.'" While the baby was in fact twenty days old, not two, this inaccuracy perhaps indicates that in the woman's eyes, regardless of the precise age, the fact that it was an infant (as opposed to an adult or even a child) is important. There exist associations of innocence, vulnerability, and pity. This immediate empathy for the infant's (and likely the infant's parents') plight despite fears of state surveillance could then represent what Nadya Pittendrigh terms intrabody resonance: "the tendency of our bodies to resonate in sympathy with one another" (2022, 88).

Finally, Edbauer's (2005) concept of rhetorical ecologies helps one see how the ban could be interpreted as a fluid exchange, an amalgamation of feelings and discourses not bound to concrete categories of audience, text, and rhetor. In fact, Edbauer likens this ecology to a virus, noting that a rhetoric is not contained by the aspects comprising its situation, such as audience and exigence, but "emerges already infected by the viral intensities that are circulating in the social field" (14).

The pre-existing anti-Muslim sentiment—the numerous discourses about the potentially harmful qualities Muslims are said to embody—exemplifies Edbauer's (2005) theory of such emergence and circulation. These feelings and conversations did not suddenly arise during the pandemic but were materializing and spreading for many years. The rhetorics were held together "trans-situationally" (Edbauer 20). For instance, UMLSHRC (2021) describes extremist Buddhist monks' accusations about all Muslims being connected to Wahhabism: a Sunni Islamic revivalist and fundamentalist movement. The UMLSHRC report states that such accusations were part of an Islamophobic campaign escalating in 2009 after the violent end of the country's decades-long civil war, further heightened after the country's 2019 Easter bomb attacks (reportedly by Islamic State-related extremists). Saroor (2020) notes that after the Easter bombings, a ban on face-veils—which had played no role in the attacks—"made every Muslim a perceived outsider." Rumors spread unchecked that restaurants run by Muslims were providing poisoned food and that Muslim doctors were sterilizing Sinhala women. Numerous Muslim men were rounded up under Emergency Regulations and the Prevention of Terrorism Act, simply for owning Qurans or notebooks with Arabic script.

[4] A tag like "right" or "isn't it" in "you know, right/isn't it?," used in Sri Lankan English.

[5] An expression used to indicate sympathy for someone, directly translated from the Sinhala word "pau."

Saroor also recalls anti-Muslim sentiment that propelled riots and mob violence in Aluthgama and Dharga Town in 2014, and in the Kandy district in 2018.[6]

This long line of racist acts against Sri Lanka's Muslims preceding the ban, then, strongly suggests that some groups had their own exigence or "need" for supporting the ban. As Edbauer notes, though various rhetorics overlap through a kind of "shared contagion" (a particularly apt metaphor in this case), the exigences themselves may differ (18).

A "Unique Pandemic Trauma"

As has been widely recognized, in a health crisis like a pandemic, issues regarding discriminated access inevitably arise. Quinn and Kumar (2014) study the Global Health Security Agenda and consider the role of international partners in grappling with health inequalities, including unequal access to care and resources. Craig draws on Sontag's work to discuss how COVID-19 marginalized already oppressed groups in terms of race, place, and class, making them doubly Othered. Similarly, Knoblauch and Moeller comment on how, with the COVID-19 pandemic, decisions were being made across the world about who received scarce medical equipment and who did not. They note that "bodies considered non-normative are deemed more expendable…Horrifically, alarmingly, this virus keeps reminding us that, as they always have, bodies matter in material and mortal ways" (2022, 16).

Sri Lanka's burial ban, however, presented a special case of discrimination. It engendered a "unique pandemic trauma" (Slater and Fonseka), utilizing a global health crisis for discrimination in very purposeful ways. And while the Bitzerian understanding of the rhetorical situation supports the view that this health crisis necessitated the ban, other approaches challenge the objective presence of such risk. In the Bitzerian view, this urgency was a given. The danger of the virus spreading through water was real and had to be managed via the ban. But Vatz's theory of the rhetorical situation as myth—as not existing apart from the rhetor's perspective and

[6] It is important to note, however, that civil society has worked extensively to build bridges and secure minority rights. As UMLSHRC observes (2021), communities have come together after the escalation of religious attacks to oppose extremism, to address other common issues including sexual and gender-based violence, to help ensure the implementation of post-conflict transitional justice measures, and to identify early warning systems to prevent future conflict.

interpretation (and I would add, articulation) of it—challenges this understanding. So does Biesecker's proposition, which shifts one's attention to the unfixed nature of the audience, and Edbauer's (2005) "rhetorical ecologies," emphasizing the amalgamated and gradual audience-text-speaker processes involved in an event. These latter theories then help understand how crises like illness, and even death, may not simply "exist" but be reacted towards and (mis)used in various ways. The apparent diffusion of a virus may, in fact, be linguistically created, instigating diverse reactions, identities, and relationships.

This rhetorical framework also helps approach the embodiment of the Muslim population through the ban. By prohibiting the burial of COVID-19 victims and labeling it a grave risk, various meanings became attached to the Muslim body. The ban framed Muslims, for whom burial is compulsory, as potentially non-conforming, those seeking special allowances, creators of problems, and health hazards. Both past and present prejudices against Muslims were infused into the process. The ban created audiences who believed in the risk discourse, audiences who did not believe but used the discourse for discrimination, and anti-audiences who rejected the discourse for scientific reasons, anti-racist reasons, or both. And while it is the government that officially initiated the ban, the varied responses to it by both individuals and groups, and the circulating narratives in the country about Muslims, merged speaker, text, and audience. The situation became an ecology of violence.

This violence becomes even clearer when considering Fleckenstein et al.'s three major categories of violence: direct, structural, and cultural (qtd. in Scot Barnett [2022]). Direct violence refers to acts that other people can witness and often includes physical, emotional, and sexual violence. Structural violence—institutionalized or institutionally sanctioned violence—is less visible than direct violence but can be implicated as a motive for direct violence. Cultural violence occurs symbolically, with aspects like language and empirical science being used to sanction structural and direct violence. Through its devastating effects on Sri Lanka's Muslim community—on the community's body-mind-spirit—the ban either directly or indirectly encompassed all three types of violence. It made evident that Muslim bodies are owned by the state, even in death.

Lastly, the ban not only harmed already dead bodies and inflicted significant emotional violence on the living; it most likely (and ironically) also generated further deaths. Many sources argue that the ban would have discouraged COVID-positive Muslims from seeking treatment, since cremation was compulsory for the disease's victims. Considering the disproportionate number of COVID-related deaths among the Muslim population, this conclusion does not appear off the mark. In fact, writing in May 2020, Saroor warns the public of a very similar issue. She notes that media portrayals of Muslims as the carriers and spreaders of the virus would (besides creating a picture of Muslims as unpatriotic and untrustworthy) alienate Muslims further and stop them from voluntarily reporting cases. By framing burial as dangerous, then, the ban not only shaped bodies presumed to be non-conforming as a threat; the ban also carried for the Muslim community, material, and potentially fatal, consequences.

Acknowledgements The idea for this topic came from a short paper I did for the course *Rhetoric: Renaissance to 20th Century* at the Department of English, The Ohio State University. I gratefully acknowledge the discussions we had in that course, and especially the feedback on my short paper given by the course professor Dr. James Fredal. I am also very grateful for the reviewers' immensely helpful comments on earlier versions of this chapter and for the editors' support.

Bibliography

Al-Dawoody, Ahmed, and Oran Finegan. "COVID-19 and Islamic Burial Laws: Safeguarding Dignity of the Dead." *Humanitarian Law & Policy*, 30 Apr. 2020, https://blogs.icrc.org/law-and-policy/2020/04/30/covid-19-islamic-burial laws/#:~:text=While%20Islamic%20law%20provides%20that,disasters%2C%20 collective%20graves%20are%20permitted.

Amarasiri. Comment on "Issue Of 'Corona' Cremations: Mr President, Please Respect The Wishes Of Muslims!" *Colombo Telegraph*, 26 March 2020, https://www.colombotelegraph.com/index.php/issue-of-corona-cremations-mr-presidentplease-respect-the-wishes-of-muslims/. Accessed 9 July 2022.

Amnesty International Public Statement. *Increased Marginalization, Discrimination and Targeting of Sri Lanka's Muslim Community*, Amnesty International, 19 Mar. 2021, https://www.amnesty.org/en/documents/asa37/3866/2021/en/.

Barnett, Scot. "Violence and Beneficence in the Rhetorics of Touch." *Bodies of Knowledge: Embodied Rhetorics in Theory and Practice*, edited by A. Abby Knoblauch and Marie E. Moeller, UP of Colorado, 2022, pp. 23–42.

Biesecker, Barbara A. "Rethinking the Rhetorical Situation from within the Thematic of 'Différance'." *Philosophy & Rhetoric*, 1989, pp. 110–130.

Bitzer, Lloyd F. "The Rhetorical Situation." *Philosophy & Rhetoric*, 1968, pp. 1–14.

Coleman Brown, Lerita. "Stigma: An Enigma Demystified." *The Disability Studies Reader*, edited by Lennard J. Davis, 4th edition, Routledge, 2013, pp. 147–162.

"Coronavirus: UK Amends Emergency Bill that called for Mandatory Cremations." *Middle East Eye*, 23 Mar. 2020. https://www.middleeasteye.net/news/coronavirus-uk-amends-emergency-bill-muslims-jews-other-faiths-mandatory-cremations.

"Covid-19: Sri Lanka Forcibly Cremates Muslim Baby Sparking Anger." *BBC News*, 26 Dec. 2020, https://www.bbc.com/news/world-asia-55359285.

Craig, David. "Pandemic and its Metaphors: Sontag Revisited in the COVID-19 Era." *European Journal of Cultural Studies*, vol. 23, no. 6, 2020, pp. 1025–1032, https://doi.org/10.1177/1367549420938403.

Cressman, Jodi, and Lisa DeTora. Introduction. *Graphic Embodiments: Perspectives on Health and Embodiment in Graphic Narratives*, edited by Lisa DeTora and Jodi Cressman, Leuven UP, 2021, pp. 13–20.

Dawood, S., et al. "Memorandum on the Disposal of Bodies of COVID-19 Victims." 2020, Available at SSRN 3739723, https://www.academia.edu/44628274/MEMORANDUM_ON_THE_DISPOSAL_OF_BODIES_OF_COVID_19_VICTIM.

Dolmage, Jay Timothy. *Disability Rhetoric*. Syracuse UP, 2014.

Edbauer, Jenny. "Unframing Models of Public Distribution: From Rhetorical Situation to Rhetorical Ecologies." *Rhetoric Society Quarterly*, vol. 35, no. 4, 2005, pp. 5–24, https://doi.org/10.1080/02773940509391320.

Ethirajan, Anbarasan. "Sri Lanka's Muslims 'Demonised' After Easter Bombings." *BBC News*, 13 Aug. 2019, https://www.bbc.com/news/world-asia-49249146.

Finegan, Oran, et al. "International Committee of the Red Cross (ICRC): General Guidance for the Management of the Dead related to COVID-19." *Forensic Science International: Synergy*, vol. 2, 2020, pp. 129–137, https://doi.org/10.1016/j.fsisyn.2020.03.007.

Knoblauch, A. Abby, and Marie E. Moeller. Introduction. "Bodies, Embodiment, Embodied Rhetorics." *Bodies of Knowledge: Embodied Rhetorics in Theory and Practice*, edited by A. Abby Knoblauch and Marie E. Moeller, UP of Colorado, 2022, pp. 3–19.

Mahmud, Haaris. "Issue of 'Corona' Cremations: Mr. President, Please Respect the Wishes of Muslims!" *Colombo Telegraph*, 26 Mar. 2020, https://www.colombotelegraph.com/index.php/issue-of-corona-cremations-mr-president-please-respect-the-wishes-of-muslims/.

Marsoof, Althaf. "The Disposal of COVID-19 Dead Bodies: Impact of Sri Lanka's Response on Fundamental Rights." *Journal of Human Rights Practice*, vol. 13, no. 3, 2022, pp. 669–689, https://doi.org/10.1093/jhuman/huab030

Meinhof, Marius. "Othering the Virus." *Discover Society*, 21 Mar. 2020, https://archive.discoversociety.org/2020/03/21/othering-the-virus/.

Perera, Lanka. Comment on "Issue Of 'Corona' Cremations: Mr President, Please Respect The Wishes Of Muslims!" *Colombo Telegraph*, 28 March 2020, https://www.colombotelegraph.com/index.php/issue-of-corona-cremations-mr-president-please-respect-the-wishes-of-muslims/. Accessed 9 July 2022.

Pittendrigh, Nadya. "The Role of Intrabody Resonance in Political Organizing." *Bodies of Knowledge: Embodied Rhetorics in Theory and Practice*, edited by A. Abby Knoblauch and Marie E. Moeller, UP of Colorado, 2022, pp. 89–104.

Price, Margaret. "The Bodymind Problem and the Possibilities of Pain." *Hypatia*, vol. 30, no. 1, 2015, pp. 268–284.

Quinn, Sandra Crouse, and Supriya Kumar. "Health Inequalities and Infectious Disease Epidemics: A Challenge for Global Health Security." *Biosecurity and Bioterrorism: Biodefense Strategy, Practice, and Science,* vol. 12, no. 5, 2014, pp. 263–273, https://doi.org/10.1089/bsp.2014.0032.

"Rhetorical Situations." The Purdue OWL, Purdue University Writing Lab, 2022. https://owl.purdue.edu/owl/general_writing/academic_writing/rhetorical_situation/index.html.

Ronnie. Comment on "Issue Of 'Corona' Cremations: Mr President, Please Respect The Wishes Of Muslims!" *Colombo Telegraph*, 26 March 2020, https://www.colombotelegraph.com/index.php/issue-of-corona-cremations-mr-presidentplease-respect-the-wishes-of-muslims/. Accessed 9 July 2022.

Saroor, Shreen. "Scapegoating the Muslims: From Aluthgama to Post-Easter Sunday to COVID 19." *Economynext*, 14 May 2020, https://economynext.com/scapegoating-the-muslims-from-aluthgama-to-post-easter-sunday-to-covid-19-69929/.

Shaheed, Ahmed et al. "Sri Lanka: Compulsory Cremation of COVID-19 Bodies Cannot Continue, say UN Experts." United Nations Office of the High Commissioner for Human Rights. *Relief Web*, Jan. 25 2021. https://www.ohchr.org/en/press-releases/2021/01/sri-lanka-compulsory-cremation-covid-19-bodies-cannot-continue-say-un.

Siddiqui, Jumaina and Melissa Nozell. "Two Years After Easter Attacks, Sri Lanka's Muslims Face Backlash." *United States Institute of Peace*, 29 Apr. 2021, https://www.usip.org/publications/2021/04/two-years-after-easter-attacks-sri-lankas-muslims-face-backlash.

Slater, Joanna, and Niha Masih. "As the World Looks for Coronavirus Scapegoats, Muslims are Blamed in India." *The Washington Post*, 23 Apr. 2020, https://www.washingtonpost.com/world/asia_pacific/as-world-looks-for-coronavirus-scapegoats-india-pins-blame-on-muslims/2020/04/22/3cb43430-7f3f-11ea-84c2-0792d8591911_story.html.

Slater, Joanna, and Piyumi Fonseka. "In Sri Lanka, a Unique Pandemic Trauma: Forced Cremations." *The Washington Post*, 12 Feb. 2021. https://www.washingtonpost.com/world/asia_pacific/sri-lanka-cremations-covid/2021/02/12/b97719a6-6562-11eb-bab8-707f8769d785_story.html.

"Small Fear whether the Dead Bodies with the Virus can be used as Biological Weapons – Dr. Channa Perera tells BBC." *Lanka Leader*, 16 Apr. 2020, https://english.theleader.lk/news/690-small-fear-whether-the-dead-bodies-with-the-virus-can-be-used-as-biological-weapons-dr-channa-perera-tells-bbc.

Sontag, Susan. *AIDS and its Metaphors*. Farrar, Straus and Giroux, 1989.

"Sri Lanka Finally Lifts Ban on Burial of COVID Victims." *Al Jazeera*, 26 Feb. 2021, https://www.aljazeera.com/news/2021/2/26/sri-lanka-finally-lifts-ban-on-burial-of-covid-victims.

"Sri Lanka's Cremation of COVID Dead a 'Human Rights Violation'." *Al Jazeera*, 25 Jan. 2021, https://www.aljazeera.com/news/2021/1/25/forced-cremations-during-pandemic-a-violation-of-human-rights-un.

Srinivasan, Meera. "Sri Lanka's Youngest Virus Victim Heightens Campaign Against Forced Cremations." *The Hindu*, 14 Dec. 2020, https://www.thehindu.com/news/international/sri-lankas-youngest-virus-victim-triggers-campaign-against-forced-cremations/article33330573.ece.

Swacha, Kathryn Yankura. "'Bridging the Gap between Food Pantries and the Kitchen Table': Teaching Embodied Literacy in the Technical Communication Classroom." *Technical Communication Quarterly*, vol. 27, no. 3, 2018, pp. 261–282, https://doi.org/10.1080/10572252.2018.1476589.

Titchkosky, Tanya. *Reading and Writing Disability Differently: The Textured Life of Embodiment*. U of Toronto P, 2020.

University of Minnesota Law School Human Rights Clinic. *Responses to Questionnaire for Report on Anti-Muslim Hatred and Discrimination*. Office of the High Commissioner for Human Rights, 2021, https://www.ohchr.org/Documents/Issues/Religion/Islamophobia-AntiMuslim/Civil%20Society%20or%20Individuals/HRLitigationandInternationalLegalAdvocacyClinicMinnesota.pdf.

U.S. Department of State. Bureau of Human Rights, Democracy, and Labor. *2018 Report on International Religious Freedom: Sri Lanka*. Office of International Religious Freedom, https://www.state.gov/reports/2018-report-on-international-religious-freedom/sri-lanka/#:~:text=The%20U.S.%20government%20estimates%20the,Muslim%2C%20and%207.4%20percent%20Christian.

Vatz, Richard E. "The Myth of the Rhetorical Situation." *Philosophy & Rhetoric*, 1973, pp. 154–161.

Wilkerson, Abby. "Embodiment." *Keywords for Disability Studies*, edited by Rachel Adams, et al., NYU Press, 2015, pp. 67–70.

Yousuf, Shereen, and Bernadette Calafell. "The Imperative for Examining Anti-Muslim Racism in Rhetorical Studies." *Communication and Critical/Cultural Studies*, vol. 15, no. 4, 2018, pp. 312–318, https://doi.org/https://doi.org/10.1080/14791420.2018.1533641.

Vaccinated by the Blood: Antiabortion Mobilization of the COVID Body

Jeannie Ludlow

Introduction

As the chapters in this volume demonstrate, the ability to envision embodiment—to represent bodies and their experiences in ways that allow us to imagine those bodies as real and relatable while simultaneously "pushing back against" the idea of "a singular body" (Spatz 2019, 14)—reminds us that bodies matter, that embodied experiences are a form of knowledge. Embodied experience, as Stephanie Hilger writes in the forward to this volume, is always liminal and changing. Embodiment, abstract understanding emerging out of embodied experiences, reflects an imbrication of the Imaginary, preceding language and rationality, with the Symbolic, reifying cultural and textual knowledges. The power of these partialities—change, liminality, imbrication—inhere in the distinction and the relationship between embodiment and the body. Ben Spatz explains that while embodiment often "carr[ies] assumptions of individuality and

J. Ludlow (✉)
Eastern Illinois University, Charleston, IL, USA
e-mail: jludlow@eiu.edu

J. Cressman et al. (eds.), *Envisioning Embodiment in the Health Humanities*, Sustainable Development Goals Series,
https://doi.org/10.1007/978-3-031-49807-7_13

biologism," it in fact is better understood as "an excess of the body" and the body as "a derivative of embodiment" (14). At the same time, as Sarah Combellick-Bidney and Arianna Genis remind us, embodiment and embodied theory rest on a conviction that "the stuff of bodies (tissues, substance, materiality) ... matter" 2018, (46). These complex relationships were concretized for me on December 1, 2021. On that day, in the midst of (and in spite of) a global pandemic, hundreds of us gathered in Washington DC in front of the steps of the Supreme Court of the United States, as the justices inside heard arguments in *Dobbs* v. *Jackson Women's Health Services*, the case that ultimately effected the dismantling of federal abortion rights by overturning *Roe* v. *Wade*.

Political rallies are, by definition, embodied. Ralliers' bodies, assembled together, represent both collective electoral power and the implications of political decisions in individuals' lives. Rallies for and against abortion rights have historically relied on a poetics of embodiment. A prochoice rally is a feminist event representing a collective call for an end to patriarchal control over reproductivity (undeniably an embodied experience) even when individual ralliers do not embrace feminism. Prochoice ralliers use their bodies to represent the agency of individual pregnant persons to make decisions involving their bodies. A prolife rally is a collective statement of support for hegemonic conservativism and the patriarchal status quo. Prolife ralliers represent the future embodiment of the fetus—signaled either positively through images of unborn babies in utero or negatively in images of dismembered fetal bodies—as well as social control over the sexual and reproductive actions of individual women and persons with the capacity for pregnancy. In both types of rally, the bodies of ralliers carry both Symbolic and Imaginary significance as they reinscribe movement norms (Allan 2014, 43, 53, 61). This chapter analyzes the prolife counterprotest to the prochoice rally at the US Supreme Court on December 1, 2021, as I experienced it that day, in order to demonstrate the ways the protest simultaneously reified the reproductive poetics of embodiment and introduced new facets of embodiment inspired by the COVID pandemic.

At the Rally: From Fetal Embodiment to COVID Embodiment

My experience of the rally and counterprotest is by no means objective, and my analysis is shaped by both my positionality as a 60-year-old, upper-middle-class, educated, white, heterosexual ciswoman and my experiences as a former abortion patient and abortion care worker. In many ways, the *Dobbs* v. *Jackson* rallies were typical of other prochoice-prolife demonstrations I have attended. The prochoice rally featured signs, T-shirts, and speeches proclaiming individual bodily integrity and positing the morality of abortion; indeed, I carried a sign that said "I had an abortion" and wore a tunic covered with the repeated phrase "[heart] abortion." Many of the prolife counterprotest signs featured huge representations of fetuses *in utero* and dismembered fetal bodies and reminded us all to think of the "other body" too, implying that an argument for the rights of someone who is pregnant by definition disregards the body gestating within that pregnant body. There were speeches, noisemakers, shouts, songs, and drumming from both groups. Around the rally site stood a perimeter of police officers, watching and occasionally reminding people that we needed to stay off the courthouse steps: our collective embodiment may have enacted Symbolic power, but individually, we were denied access to even the portico of the law (building) of the Father.

In other ways, the December 1, 2021, rally and counterprotest were very different from previous demonstrations I have attended. For one thing, there was far more intermingling of prochoice and prolife folks than is usual, a difference that eventually played a major role in the demonstration's trajectory. Typically, when such rallies are at government buildings, the two sides are cordoned off from one another. In Washington DC, this often takes the form of movable metal dividers—like the ones used by insurrectionists on January 6, 2021, to assault police officers—erected into a low fence between the two sides. That day, the movable metal dividers blocked us from the courthouse steps, but there was no boundary between the prochoice rally site and the spaces claimed by antiabortion counterprotesters. This was a difference that my provider friends commented on. "They didn't separate us," one said. "This feels less safe." On my run earlier that morning, I had passed the Supreme Court Building, where I found a group of antiabortion counterprotesters apparently camping in the rally space. I was somewhat surprised by their presence. However, since the rally space had been reserved by and permitted to a coalition of prochoice organizations, I assumed the prolife protesters would be asked to move to its perimeter as the rally began. This did not happen. We demonstrated together.

The second way the December 1 demonstration was unusual was in the tone of the messaging of some of the antiabortion protesters. Several times, antiabortion signs and chants typifying prochoice perspectives caught my attention. I was not particularly surprised; antiabortion cooptation of prochoice principles has long illustrated the power of liberal messaging even while attempting to undermine it. As I experienced it, though, this cooptation was more concentrated and less careful about redefining feminist messages while using them. Several organization-branded signs proclaiming the "rights of women" were joyfully wielded by young adults dancing, singing, and drumming in the rally site. Only when I saw someone with an "Equal Rights for Women" sign arm in arm with someone holding a "Women's Rights Begin in the Womb" sign did I discern that these "rights" signs were antiabortion. I was fully aware of the decade-long trend of prolife cooptation of prochoice and feminist discourse, not just in organizations like Feminists for Life but in more mainstream strands of the antiabortion movement. Even knowing this, I was more than once briefly stymied by a feminist message on a prolife protest sign.

I focus primarily on the third way the rally and counterprotest differed from previous similar events: the rally, counterprotest, and perhaps most importantly the interactions between prochoice ralliers and prolife counterprotesters were inflected with the COVID pandemic and the political tensions surrounding it. In fact, my friend's statement, "[t]hey didn't separate us. This feels less safe," was not simply a reference to being in a crowded space with antiabortion activists, an experience she has had at her own clinics. It also referred to the fact that half the people at the crowded venue were unmasked. Many telegraphed their skepticism of the virus and/or of vaccines, as I will describe later in this chapter. Prochoice and reproductive justice advocates attending the rally were asked by the organizing committee to mask, and as far as I could tell, almost all of us did. Antiabortion folks, even those coopting feminist messaging, by and large did not. As soon as I realized this, I found it much easier to determine whether a particular "women's rights" message was prochoice or prolife—I simply looked for a mask on the face of the person wielding the message.

At the December 1, 2021, rally and counterprotest, antiabortion activists remapped onto the COVID pandemic their customary deployment of embodied potential to invoke both affective (Imaginary) and reasoned

(Symbolic) embodied responses. These strategies are not new; antiabortion activists have long used the fetal body—a body that by definition personifies potential—in their activism, sometimes going so far as to bring dead fetuses to their protests, as historian Johanna Schoen has documented (2013, 155–62). Even when not mobilizing actual fetal bodies, the prolife movement has exploited romanticized Lennart Nilsson-like unborn baby images (Cosgrove 2023) alongside exaggerated and magnified dismembered fetus images (Schoen 155). This mobilization, as Schoen explains, transforms "the originally private (fetal) bodies [into] public entities" (158), ultimately honoring neither fetus nor abortion seeker. The prolife movement's rhetorical envisioning and fetishization of the fetal body weaponizes embodied potential, leaning on the imbrication of Symbolic and Imaginary, ostensibly to make the fetal body more "real" to abortion seekers and to the culture at large. These tactics expose primary movement goals: to stigmatize abortion and abortion-seekers, to win their argument by depriving others of dignity and autonomy, as many feminist scholars have demonstrated (Dubow 2011, Duden 1993, Hann and Ludlow 2021, Ludlow 2008, 2019, 2021, Newman 2006, Petchesky 1987, Schoen, Stabile 1992). At the rally and counterprotest at the US Supreme Court Building, the antiabortion activists remapped these tactics onto the COVID body, layering their denial of COVID over people's concerns about it and reframing received scientific knowledge of the virus, thereby chafing the Symbolic against the Imaginary in a cynical, destabilizing move. The effect was similar in shape to the ways the antiabortion movement has coopted feminist and liberal language and arguments: "Your mother chose life"; "Women deserve better"; and "at 14 weeks, she can suck her thumb" (which feminizes the fetus in prolife messaging). In each of these phrases, cooptation works to redefine the feminist perspective while negating liberal principles. Similarly, the antiabortion cooptation of COVID awareness attempted to redefine liberal attention to science while negating the ethics of care that undergirded our movement-wide agreement to mask.

In what remains of this chapter, I turn to four specific examples from that day, each of which participates in the remapping of antiabortion tactics onto the COVID body. I want to emphasize that this remapping does not in any way transform prolife ideology. In fact, the (putative) COVID body, it turns out, is a perfect vehicle for the aspects of antiabortion ideology that Carol Mason has identified as apocalyptic and millennialist (2002, 134). By apocalypticism, Mason means a mindset that is focused on the catastrophic destruction of the world or, more specifically, of American culture and/or Christian culture (which, according to movement norms, are basically the same culture anyway) (4). This unrelentingly hierarchical worldview is shaped by binaries, particularly those positing an "us" that is associated with purity, light, and Christianity against a "them," who embody impurity, darkness, and sin (75). Thus, it assumes that conflict is inevitable and ultimate, bringing about the end of American/Christian culture. Apocalypticism, then, inspires activists to shift from protest (which assumes a capacity to make change) to retribution ("we" become an "army of God" working to spread light over the darkness and impurity). Mason locates prolife ideology at the intersection of apocalypticism and millennialism, where abortion becomes "the worst thing" because it enacts the end of humanity (117). Millennialism invests the apocalyptic belief in the "End Times" with militarism, thereby "divest[ing] apocalypticism of passivity" (133, 131). It is an ideology that functions narratively to describe and transform the social order. Militarism is called for not because activists can change the (inevitable) future but because they are called by God to respond to those against whom they are opposed (117, 118, 133). Mason's analysis of the apocalyptic, millennialist, militarist foundations of the antiabortion movement provides the key to the movement's remapping of prolife embodiment onto the COVID body. The pandemic provided a perfect canvas on which counterprotesters could project their true preoccupation—not saving babies but making ready for the end of the world.

Masking: Coopting Embodiment

In the midst of the precautions many of us were taking against COVID, the absence of masks on counterprotesters at the rally felt portentous, simultaneously disconcerting and seductive. I had been wearing masks everywhere except at home for more than a year. The small city where I live prides itself on being progressively minded, so most people were masking in public. My students were required to mask in class. I had grown accustomed to, albeit not happy with, seeing only the top half of most people's faces. I even double-masked on the flight from Illinois to Washington DC, after reading news stories explaining the risks of contagion while flying. In the context of these daily experiences, the maskless smiles of the antiabortion protesters seemed almost wanton, reminding me of all we had lost. That this loss was enacted at a rally to protest another impending loss (and we knew it would be a loss, even if we were not yet sure how extensive of one) seemed particularly harsh.

I have given a lot of thought to the fact that the prochoice movement was masked and the prolife movement was unmasked. Superficially, of course, this makes sense; antiabortion activists are often also people who chafe against rules and regulations, which they characterize as "big government." At the same time, the trends in masking reflect a kind of inversion of generally received understandings of conservativism and liberalism. Reductively, the prolife movement purports to be focused on protection of the fetus/unborn child (even, at times, protection of the pregnant woman from the inherent "violence" of abortion), while the prochoice movement articulates commitments to liberal principles like individual freedom of choice and self-determination. Our masked protection of others, stacked up against their unmasked freedom, enacted an inversion of these trends that exposed the cynical cooptation of liberal and feminist discourses of people refusing to mask (reiterated in social media and news stories featuring conservatives shouting "My body, my choice!" as they were escorted out of retail establishments). The antiabortion refusal to mask (and envy-inducing delight in their bare faces) thus redefined liberal and feminist discourses even as it coopted them. It also made hyper visible the threat of potential contagion, a threat that prolife counterprotesters exploited on both interpersonal and mass levels.

"My Vaccine": Embodied Ambiguity

One of the ways prolife counterprotesters signaled their COVID skepticism was through messaging on signs and t-shirts. A number of the counterprotesters carried large vertical banners (maybe nine feet tall) shaped something like heraldic gonfaloni (rectangular with a triangular bottom). Many of these had messages that we had seen before (Bible verses or "God hates abortion" or "Ask me why you deserve HELL"), but a few had newer, COVID-specific messages. One banner declared both "Follow the science" and, immediately underneath, "Jesus is my vaccine." The apparent contradiction inherent in this pairing in many ways typifies the antiabortion counterprotesters' approach to the pandemic: simultaneously denying the received scientific knowledge of COVID while exploiting others' very rational concerns about it. In other words, this banner enacts the chafing of the Symbolic against the Imaginary described above. Another antiabortion banner made even more obvious the destabilizing effect of this tactic; the banner read:

DO NOT FEAR
coronavirus
vaccines
ANTIFA
BLM
death
You need to
FEAR GOD

The ambiguity in this list—Should one not fear coronavirus vaccines? Or coronavirus *nor* vaccines?—is likely a function of the shape of the banner and the size of the letters. Nonetheless the effect of the ambiguity is to destabilize both the message and the intended recipients in preparation for the restabilizing effect of the single, simple answer: "fear God."

I saw many T-shirts with similar messages. One read, "The Blood of Jesus is my Vaccine." These words were printed over a background sketch of a rough-hewn cross and under a foreground image of a syringe filled with red liquid; the text on the shirt effectively separated the cross from the syringe, even as the words signified continuity between them. In other words, "vaccinated," here, likely means *un*vaccinated as well as suggesting an alternative to vaccination. This T-shirt and others like it, then, signaled a declaration of faith and, simultaneously, a deployment of "belief" in the science behind COVID (as it was understood at the time) as a weapon against us. What interests me, however, are the larger implications for this messaging in the context of a prolife protest. These banners and T-shirts are intended to signal that faith supersedes embodiment and that those with faith will be saved (not only from COVID but from the apocalypse). At the same time, they emphasize the centrality of embodiment to prolife ideology in two ways. First, the focus on saving metaphorically connects religious salvation to the act of saving the body (not the spirit or soul) of the unborn child from abortion. Second, the cooptation of vaccination implies a threat of bodily illness as well as spiritual affliction to those they oppose. One particular encounter with an antiabortion protester shifted this threat from textual to experiential.

"I Have Covid!": Embodied Infringement

I attended the rally with several friends, all of whom own or manage abortion clinics in the United States. We were aware that the hearing inside the Supreme Court would move the US closer to the decimation of federal abortion rights and make way for increased limitations to access to abortion care. At one point, several of us left the rally space, seeking restrooms. A few blocks from the courthouse, a person wearing an antiabortion shirt and carrying a sign approached us on the sidewalk. It was pretty clear who we were: in addition to my "[heart] abortion" dress, we all wore the turquois #AbortionIsEssential hats distributed by the Center for Reproductive Rights, and we held signs of our own. We were masked in response to the COVID pandemic; he was not. As we passed him on the sidewalk, he turned his head toward us and coughed loudly, performatively, without covering his mouth. "I have COVID!" he yelled over his shoulder. We stopped and looked at each other for a moment. One of my friends shouted something (probably inappropriate) at his retreating back, and we went on to find toilets.

None of us really believed that he had COVID. More accurately, we didn't believe that he would know if he did. And my friends are, unfortunately, accustomed to far more aggressive threats than that one. Still, we were momentarily taken aback by his easy and aggressive weaponization of a viral pandemic that had killed hundreds of thousands of people by that time. His performative coughing clearly intended to ridicule us for our (apparent) acceptance of the received scientific analyses of transmission and prevention, as signaled by our masks. At the same time, his actions extended beyond simple derision. His unmasked face weakened the interpersonal borders established by social norms of widespread masking, redefining his performative coughing. Thus he inserted himself into our space, both materially and vaporously. This invasion was particularly jarring given the context of "social distancing" that had kept most of us at least six feet apart for the previous year and a half. He both refused to respect the new standards of distance and masking and deliberately and aggressively heaved his "droplets" in our direction, thereby imposing potential transmission and contagion onto our party. This infringement reminded us that at this rally, as in all rallies, the body served simultaneously to signify affect and to represent empowerment. In retrospect, I recognize how the embodied infringement enacted by his performative coughing and verbal threat presaged a collective infringement that reshaped the borders of the rally and counterprotest.

The COVID Crusade: Embodied Incursion

One of the most fascinating elements of the prolife counterprotest, in my experience, was something I've begun to think of as the antiabortion phalanx. When I arrived at the rally, I noticed that several of the counterprotesters whom I had earlier seen camping in front of the US Supreme Court Building appeared to be those holding the gonfalon-style rectangular banners described above. There were about a dozen of them holding banners, standing in a straight row of antiabortion protesters along the back edge of the rally space, facing the stage; another twenty or so protesters stood in line with them, spaced among the banners. None of these protesters were masked; several wore T-shirts or carried signs declaring their unvaccinated status or their COVID skepticism. Several of the large banners linked antiabortion thinking to COVID incredulity, as described above; the rest were fire-and-brimstone-inspired religious slogans or accusations that abortion is murder. I initially noticed this row of protesters primarily because of the COVID-related banners. An hour or so into the rally, however, I also noticed that they seemed closer to us than I had previously realized. I began to pay attention, and at one point, I noticed one of the protesters shout out, and everyone in the row moved forward a step.

Prochoice ralliers were clearly trying to avoid this close array of unmasked, shouting, COVID-doubting bodies. A while later, I glanced back toward them and noticed that the array was even closer to the stage, still in formation. It was disconcerting; it looked like something from *Game of Thrones* or a Peter Jackson movie. By the time the rally was winding down, the prolife/COVID-doubting phalanx had halved the rally space, making it difficult for prochoice ralliers to remain close enough to the stage to see and hear the scheduled speakers. Indeed, by the afternoon, my friends and I—and many other prochoice activists—had been displaced to behind the phalanx of antiabortion counterprotesters, relocated by a combination of their concerted movements and our COVID-related precaution.

Like the coughing man described above, these counterprotesters weaponized the COVID body's ambivalent significance, infusing it with both the Imaginary and the Symbolic. They exploited our prudence regarding the threat of contagion via the Imaginary: our ability to envision COVID inspired caution—perhaps even fear—of being too close to them. At the same time, they exploited our trust in medical science via the Symbolic: our acceptance of the materiality and material effects of a virus which is unseen and unsee-able. Like the coughing man, their unmasked-ness and anti-vaccination messaging weakened borders that we were trying to maintain. Their closeness to one another and to us subverted conventional wisdom regarding distancing, thereby creating a kind of collectivity, a congregation that occupied the rally space both materially and discursively.

Conclusion: Envisioning Post-Roe Embodiment

These embodied tactics effectively partitioned us, using the threat of COVID to organize the space as the counterprotesters used their bodies to maneuver our responses within the rally. But the real action that day was actually inside the US Supreme Court Building, where arguments in the case *Dobbs* v. *Jackson Women's Health Organization* (2023), strangely, mimed the very tactics being used outside. While I was figuring out that a "Women's Rights" sign held by one rallier reflected a very different underlying philosophy from a similar sign held by someone else, Associate Justice Brett Kavanaugh performed rhetorical ambiguity inside, presenting a miasmic counterargument to *stare decisis* based on imaginary alternative outcomes to landmark liberal cases. He argued, "[In] some of the most consequential and important [cases] in the Court's history, the Court overturned precedent." If, however, the Supreme Court had "adhere[d] to precedent in Brown v. Board, adhere[d] to Plessy ... the country would be a much different place." As I realized that masks were key, and that masked feminists ralliers were advocating for protectionism while unmasked antiabortion counterprotesters were shouting for freedom, Associate Justice Kavanaugh concluded, "if we think that the prior precedents are seriously wrong ... why then doesn't the history of this Court's practice ... tell us that the right answer is actually a return to the position of neutrality?" The obfuscation by which the justice claimed "neutrality" for an elimination of rights echoed the chicanery of the banner claiming that to "Follow the Science" is to accept "Jesus as [one's] vaccine."

This is not to claim that conservative justices expressed confidence in vaccines. To the contrary, Associate Justice Amy Coney Barrett briefly mobilized a popular conservative vaccine skepticism, seemingly in order to argue that "infringement on bodily autonomy" is sometimes reasonable.

While my friends and I were confronting the coughing man, who performatively shared his putative COVID with us, Associate Justice Barrett was, perhaps, providing context for her decisions not to block vaccine mandates in Indiana in August and in Maine in October (Romoser 2021). Amy Howe reported on the Indiana case in *SCOTUSblog*, explaining that a group of Indiana University students had appealed to the Supreme Court, asking the court to block the university's vaccine mandate. Howe (2021) writes, "Barrett, who is responsible for emergency appeals from Indiana, denied the students' request without comment, without seeking a response from the state, and without referring the request to the full court for a vote." While she made no comment in August, Associate Justice Barrett did seem to refer briefly to these situations during the *Dobbs* hearing; she said, "There is, without question, an infringement on bodily autonomy, you know, which we have in other contexts, like vaccines. However, it doesn't seem to me to follow that pregnancy and then parenthood are all part of the same burden" (*Dobbs*). This statement is doubly interesting. First, Barrett mentions vaccines in order to accept situational infringement on bodily autonomy. This acceptance was called for in the *Dobbs* hearing because the prochoice attorneys argued that denial of abortion was a denial of women's bodily autonomy. Rather than contradict this analysis, Barrett simply analogized the loss of abortion rights to vaccination. Thus, she was able to cut her argument two ways: she could implicitly defend her decisions to uphold vaccine mandates even as she subtly critiqued vaccines, in a nod to the conservative voter base. Second, Barrett makes an immediate rhetorical turn, shifting her comments from infringement to burden; this shift was particularly important given that *Dobbs* was expected to redefine the "undue burden" standard, which was applied to abortion rights in *Planned Parenthood of Southeastern Pennsylvania* v. *Casey* (2023). Associate Justice Barrett's acknowledgment of burdens and infringements while condoning them mirrored the cynical invocation of feminist arguments on the prolife organizations' signs. After the rally was over and we had returned to our hotel, I was struck while listening to the recording of the hearing of how often the justices and the attorneys deployed arguments characterized by internal contradictions.

Some four months after the December 1, 2021, rally, an initial draft of the *Dobbs* finding was leaked to the public. Like the coughing man, the US Supreme Court turned out to be a leaky body, performatively spewing not vapor or droplets but powerful words that went immediately viral. In the year since the *Dobbs* leak, we have watched the anti-abortion counterprotesters' tactics spread and morph across the United States. With *Roe* gone, the (temporary, as we had long feared) barriers of privacy and rights that protected abortion seekers' access to abortion care have become maneuverable, easily repurposed to suit conservative goals. In many states, the masks have come off, and conservative politicians no longer pretend to care about women and babies; the overarching goal to win the political argument has become the central focus of legislative responses to the end of *Roe* in both restrictive states and so-called haven states where abortion access is protected. State legislatures have also begun to fulfill Associate Justice Clarence Thomas's prediction that the *Dobbs* decision will change the legal landscape for other reproductive, sexual, and privacy matters: legal and civil rights for LGBTQ+ persons—and particularly for trans and nonbinary members of the community—have been rolled back or redefined. In many states, conservative advocates and politicians embrace internal contradiction, readily claiming that we should follow the science, seemingly confident that our science should lead us to their God.

The *Dobbs* decision rests on the fact that we have increasingly become a nation divided. In the wake of *Dobbs*, the prochoice movement has become a movement divided. Many of us are fighting in our home states to protect what access we still have. Others are working to legally help people around the borders and boundaries that prevent them from accessing abortion and gender-affirming medical care. Many others are working extra-legally to try to break down the barriers around sexual and reproductive health care that have been maintained over the last fifty years by a kind of unholy congregation of medical and legal regulation. In all these situations, prochoice activists and advocates are carefully maneuvering among an abundance of new—and very old—ways to envision embodiment, post-*Roe*.

Bibliography

Allan, Mallary. "Narrative Diversity and Sympathetic Abortion: What Online Storytelling Reveals about the Prescribed Norms of the Mainstream Movements." *Symbolic Interaction*, vol. 38, no. 1, 2014, pp. 42–63.

Combellick-Bidney, Sarah, and Arianna Genis. "Only Through the Body: Reproductive Justice and the Practice of Embodied Theory." *Women's Studies*, vol. 41, no. 1, 2018, pp. 44–59.

Cosgrove, Ben. "'Drama of Life Before Birth': Lennart Nilsson's Landmark 1965 Photo Essay." *Life*, n.d. https://www.life.com/lifestyle/drama-of-life-before-birth-landmark-work-five-decades-later/. Accessed 29 Apr. 2023.

"Dobbs v. Jackson Women's Health Organization." *Oyez*, n.d. www.oyez.org/cases/2021/19-1392. Accessed 27 Apr. 2023.

Dubow, Sara. *Ourselves Unborn: A History of the Fetus in Modern America.* Oxford UP, 2011.

Duden, Barbara. *Disembodying Women: Perspectives on Pregnancy and the Unborn.* Harvard UP, 1993.

Hann, Lena R. and Jeannie Ludlow. "Look Like a Provider: Representing the Materiality of the Fetus in Abortion Care Work." *Representing Abortion*, edited by Rachel Hurst, Routledge, 2021, pp. 119–30.

Howe, Amy. "Barrett Leaves Indiana University's Vaccine Mandate in Place." *SCOTUSblog*, 12 Aug. 2021, https://www.scotusblog.com/2021/08/barrett-leaves-indiana-universitys-vaccine-mandat-in-place/. Accessed 5 May 2023.

Ludlow, Jeannie. "Graphic Abortion: The Grotesque in Diane Noomin's 1990s Abortion Comics." *Feminist Formations*, vol. 31, no. 2, 2019, pp. 181–204.

———. "It's A ~~Boy!~~ borted: Visualizing the Fetus in Abortion Narratives." *Representing Abortion*, edited by Rachel Hurst, Routledge, 2021, pp. 49–60.

———. "Sometimes It's a Child *and* a Choice: Toward an Embodied Abortion Praxis." *Feminist Formations*, vol. 20, no. 1, 2008, pp. 26–50.

Mason, Carol. *Killing for Life: The Apocalyptic Narrative of Pro-Life Politics.* Cornell UP, 2002.

Newman, Karen. *Fetal Positions: Individualism, Science, Visuality.* Stanford UP, 2006.

Petchesky, Rosalind Pollack. "Fetal Images: The Power of Visual Culture in the Politics of Reproduction." *Feminist Studies*, vol. 13, no. 2, 1987, pp. 263–92.

"Planned Parenthood of Southeastern Pennsylvania v. Casey." *Oyez*, n.d. https://www.oyez.org/cases/1991/91-744. Accessed 5 May 2023.

Romoser, James. "Court Turns Away Religious Challenge to Maine's Vaccine Mandate for Health Care Workers." *SCOTUSblog*, 29 October 2021, https://www.scotusblog.com/2021/10/court-turns-away-religious-challenge-to-maines-vccine-mandate-for-health-care-workers/. Accessed 5 May 2023.

Schoen, Johanna. *Abortion After Roe.* U of North Carolina P, 2013.

Spatz, Ben. "Notes for Decolonizing Embodiment." *Journal of Dramatic Theory and Criticism*, vol. 33, no. 2, 2019, pp. 9–23.

Stabile, Carol A. "Shooting the Mother: Fetal Photography and the Politics of Disappearance." *Camera Obscura*, vol. 28, 1992, pp. 179–205.

Index[1]

[1] Note: Page numbers followed by 'n' refer to notes.

J. Cressman et al. (eds.), *Envisioning Embodiment in the Health Humanities*, Sustainable Development Goals Series,
https://doi.org/10.1007/978-3-031-49807-7

Springer Nature Customer Service Center GmbH
Europaplatz 3
69115 Heidelberg, Germany

FSC
www.fsc.org
MIX
Papier | Fördert gute Waldnutzung
FSC® C083411

Kolibri 360 GmbH
Ferdinand-Jühlke-Straße 7
99095 Erfurt, Deutschland
produktsicherheit@kolibri360.de